HER

D0512741

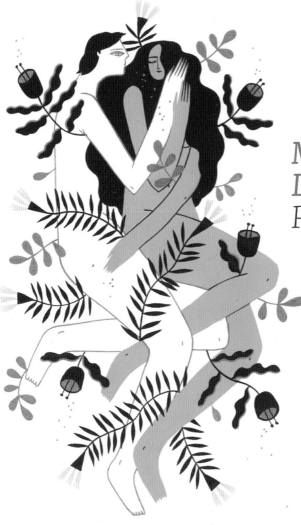

Making Love Potions

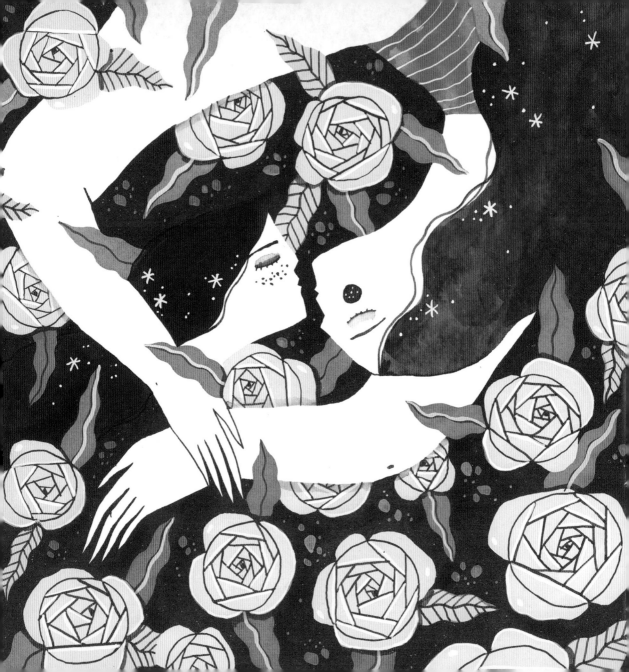

Making Love Potions

64 All-Natural Recipes for
Irresistible Herbal Aphrodisiacs

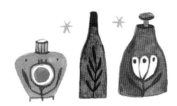

Stephanie L. Tourles

Illustrations by Madalina Andronic

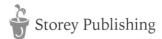

Storey Publishing

*The mission of Storey Publishing is to serve our customers by
publishing practical information that encourages
personal independence in harmony with the environment.*

Edited by Deborah Balmuth, Nancy Ringer, and Lisa H. Hiley
Art direction and book design by Jessica Armstrong
Text production by Theresa Wiscovitch
Indexed by Nancy D. Wood

Cover and interior illustrations by © Madalina Andronic
Watercolor washes throughout by © Katie Eberts
Author photograph on back cover by © Daniel Watt, Shutter Images

© 2016 by Stephanie L. Tourles

All rights reserved. No part of this book may be reproduced without written permission from the publisher,
except by a reviewer who may quote brief passages or reproduce illustrations in a review with appropriate
credits; nor may any part of this book be reproduced, stored in a retrieval system, or transmitted in any form or
by any means — electronic, mechanical, photocopying, recording, or other — without written permission from
the publisher.

The information in this book is true and complete to the best of our knowledge. All recommendations are
made without guarantee on the part of the author or Storey Publishing. The author and publisher disclaim any
liability in connection with the use of this information.

Storey books are available for special premium and promotional uses and for customized editions. For
further information, please call 800-793-9396.

Storey Publishing
210 MASS MoCA Way
North Adams, MA 01247
storey.com

Printed in Hong Kong by Great Wall Printing
10   9   8   7   6   5   4   3   2   1

Library of Congress Cataloging-in-Publication Data on file

To Shawn and summer love

Kisses from heaven
The room under the stairs
The deep silence of the cabin
Lightning bouncing across the bay
Waves lapping on the shore
Foghorns
Birch polypore incense
Tree pee
Silky, warm coconut oil
Full moon on the misty meadow
Dang blueberries
Chasing Pissah
That rogue mosquito!
Three-day musk
Bellies full of laughter
Damiana wine
Homemade clam dip & thick rippled chips
Moon-bathing on the deck as fingers of
sea smoke rose from the ocean below
A most delectable memory . . .

ACKNOWLEDGMENTS

No author writes a book alone — it takes a village, so to speak — and I would like to acknowledge and thank those who have contributed their unique fibers into the weaving of this beautiful tapestry that delves into the sensual side of herbs. First, I am especially beholden to all the men and women — friends, family, clients, fellow herbalists, acquaintances, and even total strangers — who, over the years, have shared their secrets for enkindling, exploring, and experiencing pleasurable moments with their beloved partners through the enjoyment of the senses interlaced with libido-enhancing and nourishing herbs, intoxicatingly aromatic essential oils, fragrant spices, and luscious, herb-infused foods and beverages.

Deep appreciation flows readily to Lisa Hiley and Nancy Ringer, editors extraordinaire, vocabulary masters, and "tightening professionals" with regard to reining in my profuse run-on verbiage. Somehow, in spite of having to cut thousands of my words, you two still managed to keep my "voice" and message intact! Thanks, indeed! I also wish to thank Deborah Balmuth, Storey's publisher, for offering encouragement and direction in my writing pursuits over the past two decades and giving me the opportunity to share the "sensual realm" of the herb world with my dear readers. Additionally, much gratitude goes out to the entire Storey Publishing staff — an amazing group of talented people whose support and energy have fueled the growth and strength of my career. I would not be where I am without you!

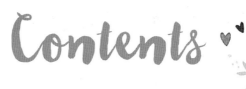

Contents

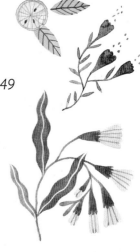

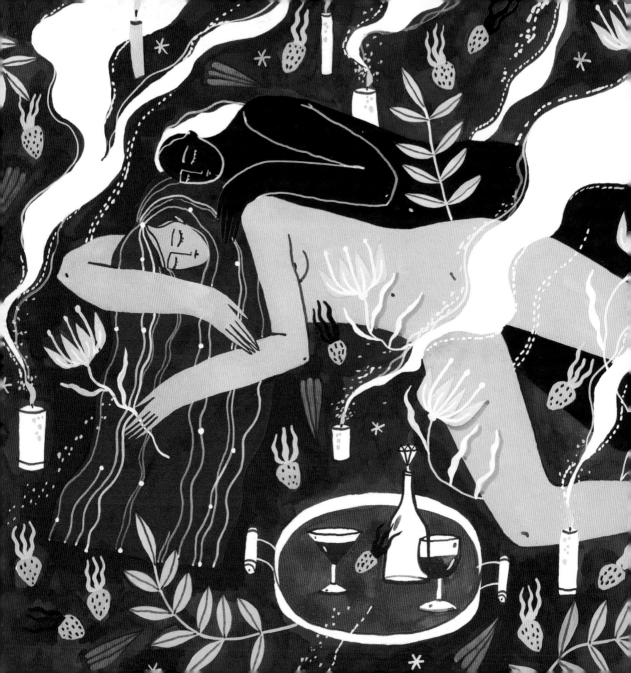

The Language of LOVE

LOVE (ENGLISH), AMORE (ITALIAN), *liefde* (Dutch), *rakkaus* (Finnish), *amour* (French), *gra* (Irish), *dragoste* (Romanian), *cariad* (Welsh), *Liebe* (German) — however you say it, love is a universal language expressed in myriad ways, through the spoken and written word, through song, by gifts of jewelry or flowers, with a smile and a wink, by dancing slowly cheek to cheek, by holding hands, by kissing, by passionate lovemaking, and sometimes simply by just being there to comfort, console, listen to, and cry with your beloved. It's a language understood by everyone. Love feels good. It is a balm for the soul. Love works magic on the human heart, quenching deep emotional, physical, and spiritual needs.

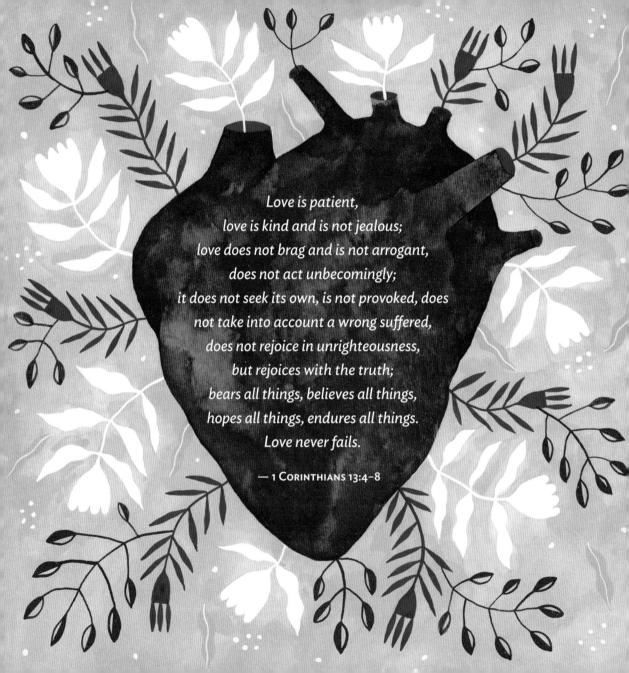

Love is patient,
love is kind and is not jealous;
love does not brag and is not arrogant,
does not act unbecomingly;
it does not seek its own, is not provoked, does
not take into account a wrong suffered,
does not rejoice in unrighteousness,
but rejoices with the truth;
bears all things, believes all things,
hopes all things, endures all things.
Love never fails.

— 1 CORINTHIANS 13:4–8

It is my own belief that a fulfilling, loving, joyful, intimate relationship between two people (whether or not it involves sexual relations) is one of the most potent and powerful healing forces in the universe. Research has, in fact, proven that positive emotions, especially the giving and receiving of love, strengthen and invigorate our immune system. On the other hand, feeling unloved or unhappy lowers our resistance to all manner of physical ailments. And people can actually die of a broken heart — such is the power of love.

But we don't always give love the care and attention it deserves. When unrelenting day-to-day stress piles up, it's easy to take our relationships for granted, to neglect those we love and put their needs on the back burner. When life gets busy and demanding, we lose sight of the importance of love — and with it all the biochemical, social-emotional, and soul-nurturing benefits it bestows upon us. So don't ignore it. Make time to pause, play, discover, rediscover, encourage, and enrich the enchantment that is love. This book can help.

The Search for the
PERFECT APHRODISIAC

From our most ancient beginnings to modern times, humans have spent a great deal of effort searching for the perfect aphrodisiac. Different cultures around the world have their own particular favored remedies, potions, and charms that are said to inspire the mood for love, invigorate sexual performance, or enhance physical sensitivity. If you look hard enough, you can probably find some folk belief proclaiming the stimulating, enticing, alluring, or seductive properties of just about any substance you can think of.

But do any of these aphrodisiacs really work? Skeptics abound, but we can't underestimate the power of those substances that relax our bodies, open our minds, excite our senses, stimulate our nerves, and thereby inspire feelings of *amore*. In fact, the arena of love offers a supremely fertile realm for the ambrosial power of herbs, fragrances, and succulent foods. Though they may never be officially approved by the Food and Drug Administration, they have time-honored, proven-in-the-real-world abilities to arouse, enhance, and energize romance and passion.

Perhaps the best aphrodisiac of all is vibrant health, physical and mental. If you're stressed out, your mind is buzzy and your body is wired. If you're tired or feeling low, your body just wants to hunker down and hibernate. Either way, your love life loses: that electric feeling of arousal wanes, and your anticipation of and pleasure in sexual activity diminishes. Here's where herbs can really shine. Some support and enhance overall good health and well-being, while others more directly target the sexual impulse.

In fact, many familiar culinary herbs such as cinnamon, ginger, nutmeg, and cayenne boost circulation, and with better blood flow to all the important regions . . . well, let's just say that these herbs spice things up in more ways than one.

Aphrodisiacs, as a category, can be different things for different people. They can stir the senses on many levels, not merely the physical, but also through scent, touch, taste . . . In short, anything that inspires or deepens the feelings of sexuality, sensuality, intimacy, joy, and contentment between you and your partner can be considered an aphrodisiac.

Herbal Effects

As just a short list, aphrodisiac herbs may

✳ Relax the mind and body

✳ Reduce nervous tension and allay the symptoms of stress

✳ Promote overall vitality and energy

✳ Improve circulation and warm the body

✳ Boost libido

✳ Support the health and function of the reproductive system

So, what is the perfect aphrodisiac? The answer will depend on the particular person. Each of us responds differently to different stimuli. To figure out what works for you and your partner, you'll have to experiment . . . and that in itself can certainly be a stimulating exploration!

Arousing Aromas

In clinical studies performed in the 1990s at the Chicago-based Smell and Taste Treatment and Research Foundation, Dr. Alan R. Hirsch examined the degree to which various scents can trigger sexual arousal in men and women, as measured by an increase in blood flow to the sexual organs. Of course, our response to scent is so much a product of our personal taste and experience that it can be hard to generalize, but it's interesting — and amusing — to note which scents elicited the largest reaction from subjects in Dr. Hirsch's study.

 SCENTS THAT TURN WOMEN ON

women's perfume	baby powder–chocolate combination	lavender–pumpkin pie combination	Good & Plenty candy–banana nut bread combination	Good & Plenty candy–cucumber combination

MILDLY AROUSING → SUPER HOT!

SCENTS THAT TURN MEN ON

women's perfume	baked cinnamon buns	cheese pizza	buttered popcorn	lily of the valley	doughnut–cola combination	licorice

MILDLY AROUSING

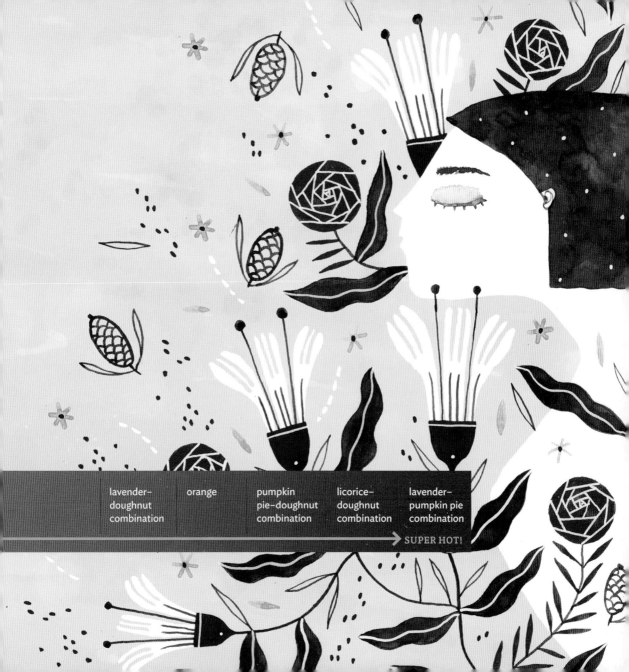

lavender–doughnut combination

orange

pumpkin pie–doughnut combination

licorice–doughnut combination

lavender–pumpkin pie combination

SUPER HOT!

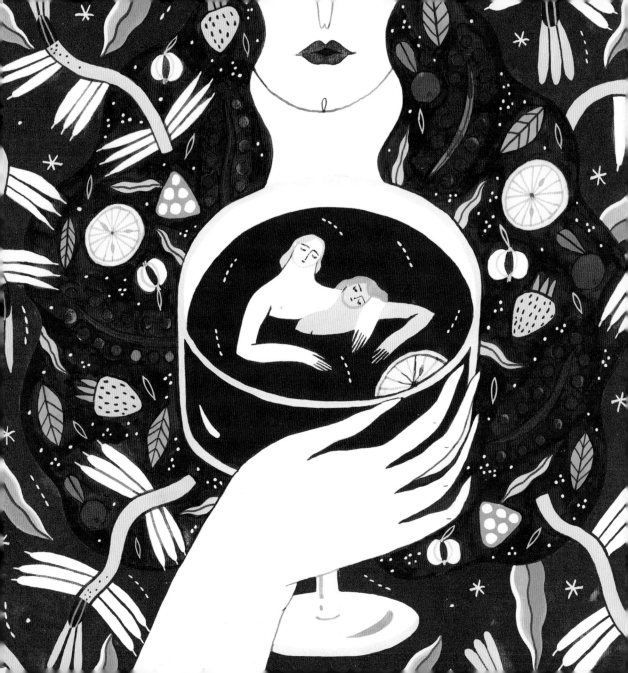

CHAPTER 1

Lascivious Libations

BEAUTIFUL TO BEHOLD, wonderfully flavored, and infused with passion-inspiring herbs, these drinks set the stage for a romantic rendezvous. There are recipes here to suit every palate, mood, and moment, whether you're looking for something thirst-quenching, revitalizing, relaxing, or warming. They make tongue-tantalizing sipping fare to share with your beloved over a romantic meal, on a blanket in front of the fireplace, or outdoors, gazing up at the stars. For special occasions or every-night delights, celebrate your love and life with a lascivious libation!

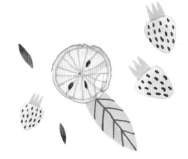

ROMANTIC RUBY-RED
Hibiscus Tea

This oh-so-tasty, slightly tart, deep red tea is perfect for Valentine's Day, birthdays, or any special occasion in which red is the color of the day and love is in the air.

INGREDIENTS

4½ cups water

2 tablespoons dried red hibiscus flowers, or 6 plain hibiscus tea bags

1 tablespoon dried lemongrass or lemon balm leaves

1 tablespoon dried rosehips

1 tablespoon dried spearmint

Honey, preferably raw (or your favorite natural sweetener)

Peel of 1 medium orange, preferably organic, cut into thin spirals (optional)

Lemon or orange slices, for garnish (optional)

Makes about 4 cups

✳ To Make

Bring the water to a boil in a medium saucepan, then remove from the heat. Add the hibiscus, lemongrass, rosehips, and spearmint, and let steep, covered, for about 45 minutes, until the tea is very deep red. Strain and add honey to taste.

✳ To Serve

Serve chilled or hot, in your most beautiful glasses or teacups, with a garnish of orange peel spiral and lemon or orange slices, if desired. Store any leftovers in the refrigerator, covered, where the tea will keep for up to 2 days.

NOTE: The Lemon Zinger and Raspberry Zinger teas from Celestial Seasonings both use hibiscus flower, and you can substitute them (use six tea bags) if you don't have plain hibiscus. A fun variation is to freeze the tea into cubes to make a flavorful and decorative addition to mixed drinks, white wine spritzers, ginger ale, or fruit punch.

Lime-Mint Fizz
WITH CRANBERRY ICE

Simply gorgeous, this sparkling, invigorating, hot pink drink is the perfect beverage to enjoy après "afternoon delight," when tasty, light refreshment is in order! The drink gets sweeter as the cranberry cubes melt, which is a most pleasant treat.

INGREDIENTS

Cranberry juice, sweetened as desired

10 fresh peppermint or spearmint leaves, or 2 drops peppermint or spearmint essential oil

Juice of 2 limes (about ⅓ cup)

Plain seltzer or sparkling water

Lime slices, fresh cranberries, or mint sprigs, for garnish (optional)

Makes 2 servings

✴ To Make and Serve

Fill two ice cube trays with cranberry juice and freeze. To prepare the drinks, you'll need two tall glasses. Finely chop the mint leaves, and divide them between the glasses (or put 1 drop of essential oil in each glass). Generously fill the glasses with cranberry ice cubes, then ever-so-slowly drizzle half of the lime juice over the ice in each glass. Top off the glasses with seltzer, and garnish with slices of lime, whole cranberries, or mint sprigs, if desired. A colorful straw is nice, too!

Variation: To make an elegant champagne cocktail, substitute champagne for the seltzer or the sparkling cranberry lemonade on the next page. It's a most beautiful party drink!

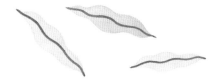

"Pucker Up" SPARKLING CRANBERRY LEMONADE

Get ready for some yummy sippin' and luscious kissin'! This gloriously red, refreshing, sweet-tart beverage is sure to delight. The bright, bold, mouth-puckering flavors of cranberries and lemons mingle, tingle, and dance on your tongue.

INGREDIENTS

- 1 cup cranberry juice, sweetened as desired
- Juice of 2 small lemons (about ⅓ cup)
- Natural sweetener of choice (raw honey, raw agave nectar, raw sugar, or stevia)
- 1½ cups plain seltzer or sparkling water
- Ice, crushed or cubed (optional)
- Lemon slices or fresh cranberries, for garnish (optional)

Makes 2 servings

✳ To Make

Combine the cranberry juice, lemon juice, and sweetener to taste in a small glass or plastic pitcher. Chill in the refrigerator for at least 2 hours to allow the flavors to meld.

✳ To Serve

Add the seltzer water to the juice blend and stir gently. Pour into two beautiful chilled glasses, filled with ice if you like. Garnish the glasses with lemon slices or a few fresh cranberries, if desired.

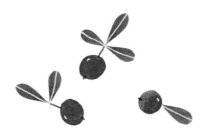

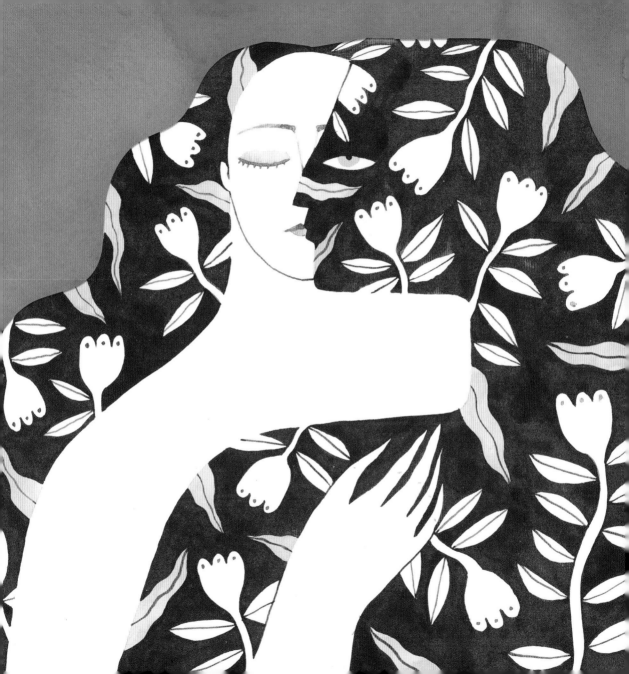

Sip 'n' Kiss TEA

This tea is sheer sensory delight. With a unique flavor that evokes a cross between homemade lemonade and natural ginger ale, with a strong minty zip, it teases and tantalizes, warms and cools, stimulates and tingles. It's perfect as an after-dinner refreshment — and it doubles as a comforting gargle for sore throats, too.

INGREDIENTS

- 2 cups water
- 1 tablespoon dried peppermint, or 3 peppermint tea bags
- 1 tablespoon freshly grated ginger
- 2 tablespoons honey, preferably raw (or your favorite natural sweetener)
- 1 tablespoon fresh lemon juice

Makes 2 servings

✳ To Make

Bring the water to a boil in a small saucepan, then remove from the heat. Add the peppermint tea bags and the ginger and let steep, covered, for 30 minutes. Strain, then stir in the honey and lemon juice.

✳ To Serve

Enjoy this zingy tea anytime your mouth needs a bit of refreshing, delicious stimulation. It's wonderful whether served over ice or piping hot.

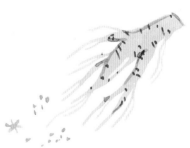

CHERRY *Kissing* CORDIAL

Gorgeously deep red, this spicy, tart-sweet cherry cordial is perfect for sipping on chilly evenings as you and your beloved revel in each other's company by a crackling fire. The cherry brandy flavor is divinely intense and warming as it dances across your tongue, making this an intriguing "kissing cordial," to say the least!

INGREDIENTS

- 1 cup good-quality 80-proof brandy
- ½ cup tart cherry concentrate
- ⅓ cup raw honey, raw agave nectar, or maple syrup
- 3 cinnamon sticks
- 6 whole allspice berries
- 1 vanilla bean, sliced lengthwise and cut into ½-inch pieces

Makes about 1¾ cups

✳ To Make

Combine the brandy, cherry concentrate, honey, cinnamon, allspice, and vanilla bean in a pint-size canning jar. Cover the jar with a piece of plastic wrap and screw on the lid. Shake the mixture vigorously for at least 15 seconds to blend. Let the cordial steep in a cool, dark place for 4 weeks, shaking the contents daily to encourage the flavors to mingle and mellow.

Strain the liquid through a fine-mesh strainer. Store in a decorative bottle, to which you've added a beautiful label, in the refrigerator and consume within 3 months.

✳ To Serve

Pour a small amount of chilled beverage into two tiny cordial cups or beautiful, slender stemware. (Or perhaps use your lover's belly button as an enticing cup from which to sip?) Because it can be quite intoxicating, consume just a bit, or you may become too relaxed to romp!

Smoldering
CHOCOLATE-VANILLA CORDIAL

A must-make beverage for the chocolate connoisseur! Oh my goodness . . . slightly bitter and nutty, gently smoky, raw, dark cacao nibs meld with warm, sweet vanilla beans to yield a sumptuous, smooth cordial with amazing depth of flavor and an aromatic intensity that just has to be experienced. This stuff makes me swoon!

INGREDIENTS

- 1¼ cups good-quality 80-proof vodka
- 1¼ cups good-quality 80-proof brandy
- ½ cup raw honey or raw agave nectar
- 2 cups raw cacao nibs
- 8 vanilla beans, sliced lengthwise and cut into ½-inch pieces

Makes about 2½ cups

✴ To Make

Combine the vodka, brandy, honey, cacao nibs, and vanilla beans in a quart-size canning jar. Cover the jar with a piece of plastic wrap and screw on the lid. Shake the mixture vigorously for 20 to 30 seconds to blend. Let the cordial steep in a cool, dark place for 8 weeks, shaking the contents daily to encourage the flavors to mingle and mellow.

Strain the liquid through a fine-mesh strainer into a decorative bottle with a beautiful label. Store in the refrigerator and consume within 3 months.

✳ To Serve

Pour a small amount of chilled liqueur into two tiny cordial cups or beautiful, slender stemware and enjoy with your lover. Aside from being quite intoxicating, this cordial also produces rather exhilarating effects from the caffeine and phenylethylamine (sometimes called the "love drug") in the raw cacao nibs, so consume in moderation until you know how it makes you feel. Personally, I like a little bit mixed with a splash of heavy cream, poured over a couple of ice cubes in a small tumbler.

Try This

For a stimulating after-dinner drink, pour 2 to 4 tablespoons of the cordial into a cup of hot coffee, add cream to taste and a dash of cinnamon or nutmeg, and you've got a delectable beverage that'll warm you right down to your toes. It's guaranteed to keep your energy soaring for a long night of passion!

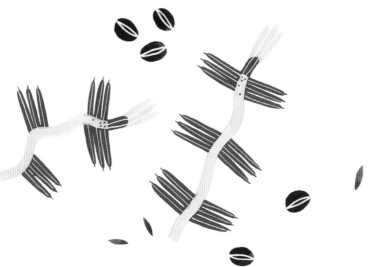

THE ORIGINS OF CORDIALS

Cordials were originally used in medieval times as medicine for various ailments and as love potions or aphrodisiacs. In fact, the word *cordial* reflects these origins. It is derived from the Latin *cor*, meaning "heart," because the earliest cordials were administered to the sick to stimulate the heart and lighten the spirit. A delicious cordial was often shared to "bring heart" to a situation, friendship, or budding romantic relationship. (In case you're wondering, yes, the terms *cordial* and *liqueur* are used interchangeably, though cordials are generally much sweeter.)

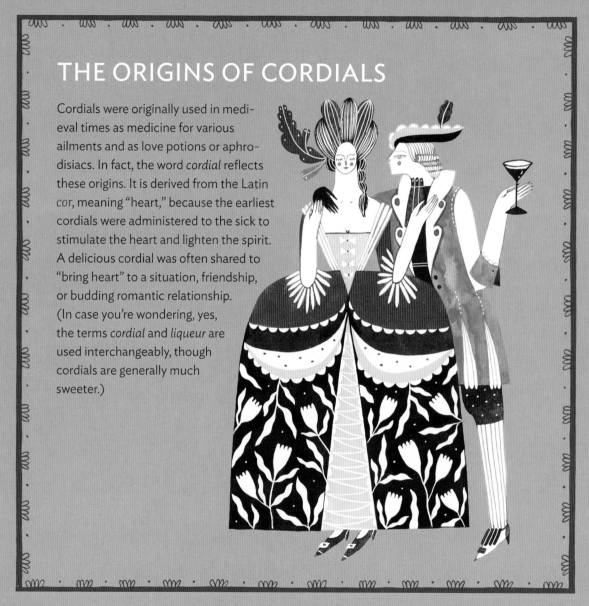

Sassy SANGRIA

A simple yet elegant drink to serve to company — perhaps your favorite couple on "double date night" at your house. It's especially wonderful when enjoyed on a warm summer's eve while sitting outside under the stars or around a fire.

INGREDIENTS

- 2 bottles fine white or red wine, preferably organic
- ½ cup diced Granny Smith apple (or another firm, semi-tart apple variety)
- ½ cup blackberries
- ½ cup blueberries
- ½ cup chopped orange, tangerine, or tangelo (peeled)
- ½ cup diced peaches
- ½ cup diced pineapple
- ½ cup raspberries
- ½ cup diced strawberries

Makes 6–8 servings

✳ To Make

Pour the bottles of wine into a pretty glass punch bowl, and add the apple, blackberries, blueberries, orange, peaches, pineapple, raspberries, and strawberries. Gently stir to mix. Cover and chill the sangria for at least 2 hours in the refrigerator prior to serving.

✳ To Serve

Ladle into chilled wineglasses, being sure to include plenty of yummy fruit bits. Drink up and savor the flavor!

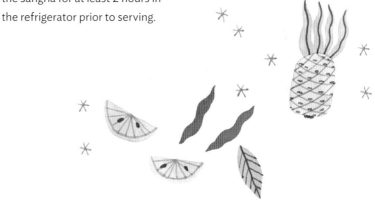

POMEGRANATE
Passion Fruit Punch

This punch is a refreshing, tart, and tangy drink with a zesty bite of ginger and a gorgeous, deep blood-red hue. And it delivers impressive amounts of energizing and immune-boosting antioxidants! Enjoy it as a delicious fruit juice blend, or ramp it up a bit by adding a splash of vodka or rum. Perfect for Valentine's Day — or any celebration of love!

INGREDIENTS

- 1 (16-ounce) bottle pure pomegranate juice
- Juice of 2 limes (about ⅓ cup)
- Juice of 1 orange or tangerine (about ⅓ cup)
- 2 teaspoons finely minced ginger
- Lime or orange slices, for garnish (optional)

Makes 2 servings

✳ To Make

Combine the pomegranate juice, lime juice, orange juice, and ginger in a small glass or plastic storage container and chill in the refrigerator for at least 2 hours to allow the zippy flavor of the ginger to infuse the juices.

✳ To Serve

Decide whether you want to strain out the ginger bits. If you leave them in (I do), just chew them as you enjoy your beverage; they freshen the breath and aid in digestion — two great benefits. Shake the punch well, and pour into two chilled glasses, with or without ice. Garnish with lime or orange slices, if desired.

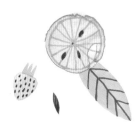

THE FRUIT OF FERTILITY

Since ancient times, the pomegranate has been hailed as a promoter of fertility. In fact, in Armenia, the pomegranate is a symbol representing marriage and abundance. The fruit was often mentioned in historical writings as having amazing health benefits, such as boosting the immune system, preserving youthful vitality, and promoting longevity, and indeed, modern research supports these claims, having shown that the pomegranate is an incredibly rich source of antioxidants.

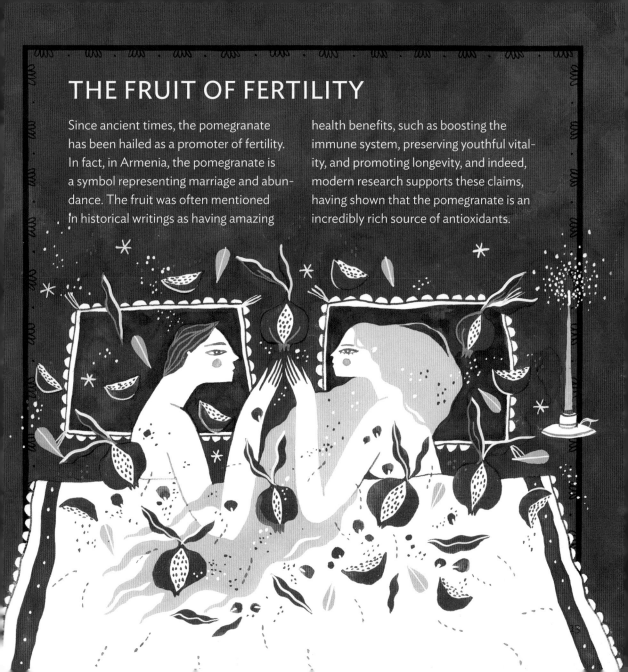

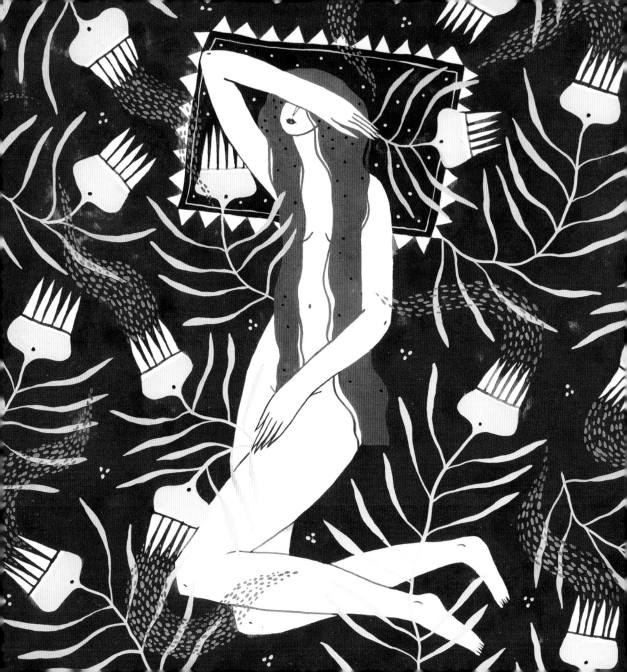

CHAPTER 2

Scentual Treasures
to Entice and Delight

OUR SENSE OF SMELL IS OUR most primitive aid to courtship, and it is willing to be seduced by an incredible range of aromas, from musky body odors to the grassy scents of various herbs, the sultry aroma of frankincense, and the sweet fragrances of flowers. Scents can soothe you, arouse you, intrigue you, remind you, alarm you, and even disgust you. They are very deeply linked to the emotions and can elicit profound physiological effects.

Following are some of my favorite recipes for evocative aromatic delights to awaken the senses, pamper the skin, stir the soul, and inspire romance. Use them to scent your own or your partner's body, your bedsheets, your home — the combination of enchanting tactile and aromatic sensations is sure to pleasure and please. And if you enjoy herbal crafting, note that many of these recipes make unique and charming handmade gifts for marriage celebrations.

Aromatic Dusting Powders

Dusting powders have a definite allure, seducing you with their silky-soft texture, subtle scent, and touch of old-fashioned elegance and grace. A well-made powder can add a little luxury and velvety smoothness to your skin that you can't get from lotions or oils alone, while keeping you dry and reducing body odor. I like to package my fragrant powders in glass shaker jars, cardboard powder tubes, antique lidded glass bowls, fancy tins, or beautiful wooden boxes. A soft powder puff makes the perfect applicator (I always keep one in my own blue glass powder bowl), though of course you can also simply shake a bit of powder into your hands and gently apply it to your chest, underarms, or any other parts you desire to pleasantly scent and keep dry.

If you've never indulged yourself with a natural body powder, please try one of these blends — I can almost guarantee that they'll soon become part of your personal fragrance collection!

Ointment and perfume rejoice the heart.

— **Proverbs 27:9**

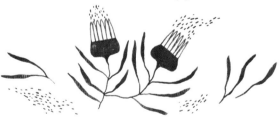

Lavender & Roses
BODY POWDER

A sweet, refined floral aroma emanates from this delicate powder. Most people adore the calming, old-fashioned fragrance of lavender — it's among the favorites for men (see Arousing Aromas, page xiv). And who doesn't love the heady scent of roses? The combination is exquisite!

INGREDIENTS

- 1 cup cornstarch or arrowroot powder, preferably organic
- ½ cup lavender flower powder
- ½ cup rose petal powder
- 50 drops geranium essential oil
- 50 drops lavender essential oil

Makes about 2 cups

✳ To Make

Combine the cornstarch, lavender powder, and rose powder in a large bowl or food processor. Gently whisk together or pulse in the food processor for 15 seconds, until well blended. Add the essential oils, drop by drop. If you're mixing by hand, whisk the mixture slowly or place the entire batch in a large container with a tight-fitting lid and shake vigorously. If you're using a food processor, pulse the mixture for another 15 seconds to thoroughly incorporate the oils. Does the powder feel nice and silky? If not, pass it through a flour sifter or sieve to remove any gritty or lumpy bits.

Store the powder in an airtight storage container in a cool, dark place for 2 weeks to allow the scent to permeate the mixture. Package the powder in smaller decorative containers, if desired, being sure to label and date each one. No refrigeration is required, but for maximum fragrance enjoyment, use within 1 year.

✳ To Use

Apply as you would any body powder, by sprinkling or using a powder puff.

Vanilla Spice
BODY POWDER

This silky powder has a round, full, sensual, spicy fragrance that appeals to both men and women. It's quite heavenly and doesn't overwhelm the senses.

INGREDIENTS

- 1¾ cups cornstarch or arrowroot powder, preferably organic
- ¼ cup baking soda
- 2 tablespoons ground cardamom
- 2 tablespoons ground cinnamon
- 2 tablespoons vanilla bean powder, or 50 drops vanilla (CO_2) essential oil
- 2 teaspoons ground cloves
- 2 teaspoons ground nutmeg

Makes about 2½ cups

✳ To Make

Combine the cornstarch, baking soda, cardamom, cinnamon, vanilla, cloves, and nutmeg in a large bowl or food processor. Gently whisk together or pulse in the food processor for 15 seconds, until well blended. If needed, pass the powder through a flour sifter or sieve to remove any gritty spice bits. Store the powder in an airtight storage container (such as a quart-size canning jar or plastic tub) in a cool, dark place for 2 weeks to allow the scent of the spices to permeate the mixture.

Package the powder in smaller decorative containers, if desired, being sure to label and date each one. No refrigeration is required, but for maximum fragrance enjoyment, use within 1 year.

✳ To Use

Apply as you would any body powder, by sprinkling or using a powder puff.

CO$_2$: SUPERIOR EXTRACTION

Sometimes you'll see the annotation "CO$_2$," after the name of an essential oil. What does it mean? Pure essential oils are extracted primarily by steam distillation, with the exception of citrus oils, which are generally cold-pressed from the fruit's rind. Occasionally petroleum solvents are used when extracting an essential oil such as jasmine, rose, or hyacinth, resulting in an "absolute" that is deemed suitable solely for fragrance, such as in natural perfumes, not for aromatherapy, as these oils retain a slight solvent residue in the final product.

A relatively new method of extraction is called supercritical carbon dioxide (CO$_2$) extraction — a more expensive yet superior process conducted under high pressure and relatively low heat without the use of steam or deleterious solvents. CO$_2$ extraction is most often used for the more expensive and oil-stingy plant materials, such as frankincense, myrrh, nutmeg, ginger, calendula blossom, and vanilla bean. When you see the designation "CO$_2$," after the name of an essential oil, it indicates that this particular essential oil has been produced via that process.

Pumpkin Pie Spice
BODY POWDER

As odd as it may sound, of all the scents that turn men on, pumpkin pie spice ranks at the top of the chart (see Arousing Aromas on page xiv for proof), and this body powder captures that comforting, relaxing, enticing aroma. Women find it alluring as well!

INGREDIENTS

1¾ cups cornstarch or arrowroot powder, preferably organic

¼ cup baking soda

8 tablespoons pumpkin pie spice

Makes about 2½ cups

✳ To Make

Combine the cornstarch, baking soda, and pumpkin pie spice in a large bowl or food processor. Gently whisk together or pulse in the food processor for 15 seconds, until well blended. If needed, pass the powder through a flour sifter or sieve to remove any gritty spice bits. Store the powder in an airtight storage container (such as a quart-size canning jar or plastic tub) in a cool, dark place for 2 weeks to allow the scent of the spice to permeate the mixture.

Package the powder in smaller decorative containers, if desired, being sure to label and date each one. No refrigeration is required, but for maximum fragrance enjoyment, use within 1 year.

✳ To Use

Apply as you would any body powder, by sprinkling or using a powder puff.

"Come Hither"
BODY POWDER

Opposites attract and here warm, resinous frankincense complements soft, sweet lavender, building up to an interesting and intriguing harmony. Together they mingle for an atmosphere that's sure to tingle. This scent smells simply divine on everyone.

INGREDIENTS

- 1 cup cornstarch or arrowroot powder, preferably organic
- ½ cup baking soda
- ½ cup lavender flower powder
- 60 drops lavender essential oil
- 35 drops frankincense (CO₂) essential oil

Makes about 2 cups

✳ To Make

Combine the cornstarch, baking soda, and lavender powder in a large bowl or food processor. Gently whisk together or pulse in the food processor for 15 seconds, until well blended. Add the essential oils, drop by drop. If you're mixing by hand, whisk the mixture slowly, or place the entire batch in a large container with a tight-fitting lid and shake vigorously. If you're using a food processor, pulse the mixture for another 15 seconds to thoroughly incorporate the oils. Does the powder feel nice and silky? If not, pass it through a flour sifter or sieve to remove any gritty or lumpy bits.

Store the powder in an airtight storage container in a cool, dark place for 2 weeks to allow the scent to permeate the mixture.

Package the powder in smaller decorative containers, if desired, being sure to label and date each one. No refrigeration is required, but for maximum fragrance enjoyment, use within 1 year.

✳ To Use

Apply as you would any body powder, by sprinkling or using a powder puff.

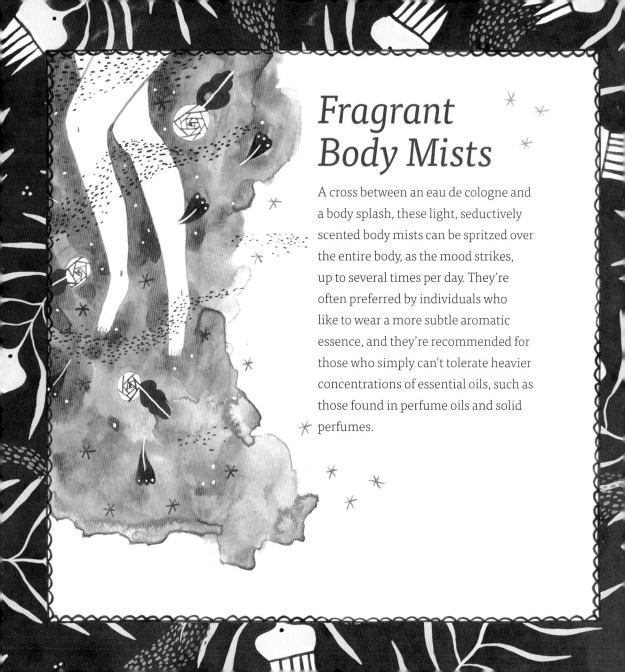

Fragrant Body Mists

A cross between an eau de cologne and a body splash, these light, seductively scented body mists can be spritzed over the entire body, as the mood strikes, up to several times per day. They're often preferred by individuals who like to wear a more subtle aromatic essence, and they're recommended for those who simply can't tolerate heavier concentrations of essential oils, such as those found in perfume oils and solid perfumes.

Mountain Man BODY MIST

Masculine and outdoorsy, reminiscent of a fresh, sweet, northern evergreen forest mingled with rich and intriguing balsamic, spice, and resinous undertones, this mist blends nicely with a man's natural musky essence, making for an interesting, enticing, and aphrodisiacal fragrance. It's wonderful when spritzed onto bed linens prior to an evening of playful passion.

INGREDIENTS

- 7 drops cedarwood essential oil
- 7 drops juniper berry essential oil
- 5 drops balsam fir essential oil
- 4 drops rosemary essential oil
- 3 drops frankincense (CO$_2$) essential oil
- 3 drops myrrh essential oil
- 2 teaspoons 80-proof vodka
- 3 tablespoons plus 1 teaspoon water

Makes about ¼ cup

✳ To Make

Combine the cedarwood, juniper berry, fir, rosemary, frankincense, and myrrh essential oils in a 2-ounce dark glass spritzer bottle. Pour in the vodka and water, screw on the top, and shake vigorously to blend. Label, then set aside for 24 hours to allow the essential oils to synergize and the fragrance to develop. Store at room temperature, away from heat and light; use within 1 year.

✳ To Use

Shake well, then spritz anywhere on your body, up to several times per day.

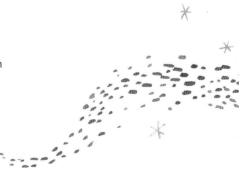

Ma Cherie BODY MIST

Smoldering, grounding, and divine, this body mist, with its blend of smooth, round, rich, slightly musky, earthy, and ethereal-floral sweet notes is simply intoxicating. A fine fragrance, indeed! It doubles as a lovely aromatic spray for the boudoir — a few spritzes on your bed linens and pillows imparts an alluring, aphrodisiacal fragrance.

INGREDIENTS

- 4 drops palmarosa essential oil
- 4 drops patchouli essential oil
- 4 drops Australian sandalwood essential oil
- 1 teaspoon natural vanilla extract, preferably made from premium Madagascar Bourbon or Tahitian vanilla beans
- 2 teaspoons 80-proof vodka
- 3 tablespoons rose hydrosol

Makes about ¼ cup

✳ To Make

Combine the palmarosa, patchouli, and sandalwood essential oils in a 2-ounce dark glass spritzer bottle. Add the vanilla extract, vodka, and rose hydrosol, screw on the top, and shake vigorously to blend. Label, then set aside for 24 hours to allow the essential oils to synergize and the fragrance to develop. Store at room temperature, away from heat and light; use within 1 year.

✳ To Use

Shake well, then spritz anywhere on your body, up to several times per day.

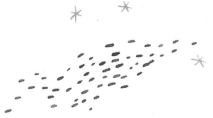

VANILLA: A FINE FRAGRANCE SECRET

The aroma of Madagascar Bourbon and Tahitian vanilla beans can be described as rich, creamy, somewhat woody-floral, and slightly musky and tobacco-like, with a deep balsamic, spicy-sweet body. When the beans are masterfully blended and aged with just the right proportions of water and alcohol (like a fine wine), a luscious, round, oh-so-fragrant vanilla extract develops, one with a scent that is familiar, comforting, and relaxing, yet sensually alluring.

This type of premium vanilla extract is highly prized as a flavoring additive (obviously), but it's also tremendously popular as a personal scent. Surprised?

Don't be. Many natural perfumers often use premium vanilla extract as a base ingredient in their formulations, as it lends a softness and warmth to any blend. You can enjoy it as a fine personal fragrance by simply dabbing a drop on several pulse points, such as inside the wrists and elbows, behind the earlobes, on the temples, at the nape of the neck, on your cleavage/sternum, under your arms, behind the knees, and on the ankles. You'll smell divinely edible! Mmm . . . think of the possibilities!

To make your own premium vanilla extract, see my recipe on page 31.

Magikal Mystique
BODY MIST

Complex, pungent, evocative, and warming, this magical pairing of two precious resins results in a deep, rich, robust essence with hints of lemon, pepper, spice, and sweet-balsamic-woody undertones that's adored by both men and women. Regarded as "base notes" in the perfumery realm, frankincense and myrrh combine to produce a long-lasting scent that mingles and mellows as the hours pass. Due to the inherent astringent properties of frankincense and, especially, myrrh, this mist doubles as a deodorizing body and foot spray.

INGREDIENTS

- 14 drops frankincense (CO_2) essential oil
- 10 drops myrrh essential oil
- 2 teaspoons 80-proof vodka
- 3 tablespoons plus 1 teaspoon water

Makes about ¼ cup

 To Make

Combine the frankincense and myrrh essential oils in a 2-ounce dark glass spritzer bottle. Pour in the vodka and water, screw on the top, and shake vigorously to blend. Label, then set aside for 24 hours to allow the essential oils to synergize and the fragrance to develop. Store at room temperature, away from heat and light; use within 1 year.

To Use

Shake well, then spritz anywhere on your body, up to several times per day.

"I Want to Kiss You All Over"
BODY MIST

Ooh-la-la! This sumptuous body mist may remind you of fresh-baked doughnuts or perhaps gently spicy snickerdoodle cookies, rich with the aromatics of vanilla bean, sweet orange, ginger, cinnamon, clove, cardamom, and allspice. Both men and women find these "comfort food fragrances" alluring, so if you want to smell delectable, spritz some on everywhere. This mist doubles as an enticing spray for the boudoir — a few spritzes on your bedding and pillows imparts a deeply intriguing, aphrodisiacal fragrance.

INGREDIENTS

- 8 drops sweet orange essential oil
- 4 drops ginger essential oil
- 3 drops cinnamon bark essential oil
- 3 drops clove essential oil
- 2 drops allspice essential oil
- 2 drops cardamom essential oil
- 2 tablespoons vanilla extract, preferably made from Madagascar Bourbon or Tahitian vanilla beans
- 2 tablespoons water

Makes about ¼ cup

✳ To Make

Combine the sweet orange, ginger, cinnamon, clove, allspice, and cardamom essential oils in a 2-ounce dark glass spritzer bottle. Pour in the vanilla extract and water, screw on the top, and shake vigorously to blend. Label, then set aside for 24 hours to allow the essential oils to synergize and the fragrance to develop. Store at room temperature, away from heat and light; use within 1 year.

✳ To Use

Shake well, then spritz anywhere on your body, up to several times per day.

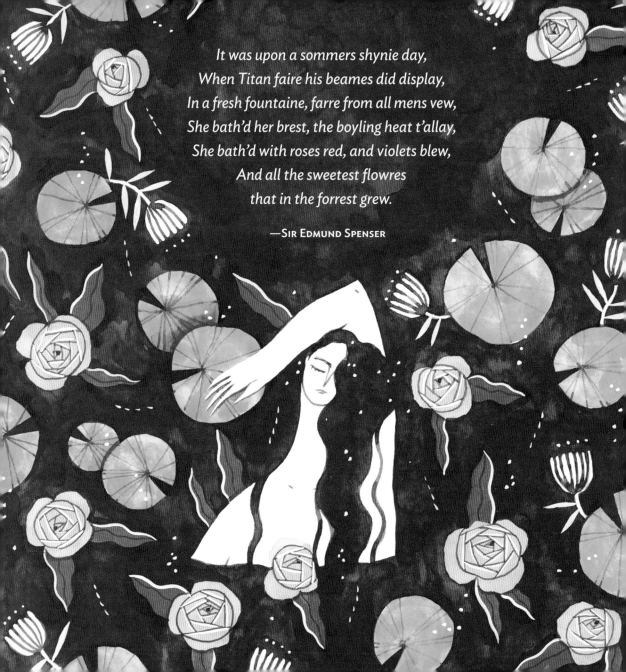

It was upon a sommers shynie day,
When Titan faire his beames did display,
In a fresh fountaine, farre from all mens vew,
She bath'd her brest, the boyling heat t'allay,
She bath'd with roses red, and violets blew,
And all the sweetest flowres
that in the forrest grew.

—SIR EDMUND SPENSER

"My Precious"
ESSENCE OF ROSE BODY MIST

Fresh, light, sensuous, and subtle, this is one of my most favored aromatic body mists. It combines the essence of true rose with the gentle spicy-green overtones of rose geranium. If you want a relatively inexpensive way to use rose as your personal fragrance, then make this mist.

INGREDIENTS

- ¼ cup rose hydrosol
- ¼ cup rose geranium hydrosol
- 2 drops geranium essential oil

Makes about ½ cup

✳ To Make

Combine the rose hydrosol, rose geranium hydrosol, and geranium essential oil in a 4-ounce dark glass spritzer bottle. Screw on the cap and shake vigorously to blend. Label, then set aside for 24 hours to allow the fragrance to synergize and develop. Store in a dark, cool cabinet; use within 1 year.

✳ To Use

Shake well, then spritz anywhere on your body, up to several times per day.

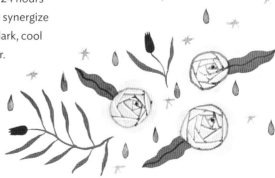

Vanilla Lover's LINEN SPRAY

Love all things vanilla? I do, and so do many women and men. The familiar rich, sweet scent is a softly seductive fragrance to spray on your bed linens for an inviting atmosphere. It's sure to pleasure and please in a most delicious way! The spray doubles as a lingering, sensual body and hair mist that can be spritzed on anytime you desire. For the vanilla, use an extract made from premium Madagascar Bourbon or Tahitian vanilla beans or make your own (see facing page).

INGREDIENTS

2 tablespoons
   vanilla extract

2 tablespoons
   purified water

Makes about ¼ cup

✳ To Make

Add the vanilla extract and water to a 2-ounce dark glass spritzer bottle, screw on the top, and shake vigorously to blend. Label, then set aside for 24 hours to allow the blend to mellow. Store at room temperature, away from heat and light; use within 1 year.

✳ To Use

Shake well, then lightly spritz sheets and pillowcases a few minutes prior to your romantic encounter.

DIY: *Sumptuous Vanilla Extract*

Like many crafty home cooks, I prefer to make my own vanilla extract. It's easy and economical, and the resulting dark, velvety extract has an incredibly rich, creamy, full, round flavor and aroma that are simply out of this world! For the alcohol I use Captain Morgan Original Spiced Rum, which makes a wonderful complement to the vanilla beans, but you can substitute any good-quality brandy, unflavored vodka, bourbon, or plain rum.

To make the extract, all you need is the following:

* 8 whole vanilla beans (make sure they're fresh and smell strongly of vanilla)

* 2 cups Captain Morgan Original Spiced Rum

* Pint-size canning jar with lid

* Plastic wrap

Slice each vanilla bean lengthwise and chop into tiny pieces. Add the vanilla bean bits to a pint-size canning jar, then fill the jar with the rum. Place a piece of plastic wrap over the top of the jar and screw on the lid. Shake for 1 minute.

Store the jar in a dark cabinet for 2 months, shaking daily for 10 to 15 seconds. There's no need to strain out the bean bits; just leave them in the jar. The flavoring will get stronger and even more aromatic as it ages. It smells so good that I sometimes dab it on as perfume!

Irresistible Perfume Oils

Perfume oils are heavier than alcohol- and water-based cologne sprays or body mists (see page 22), which tend to evaporate comparatively quickly. Their aroma sinks right into your skin and lingers, developing and blooming as the hours pass.

For oil-based perfumes, I prefer to use jojoba oil as the base because it does not become rancid over time, meaning that your perfume oils will last a long time, and because it is chemically similar to human sebum (the natural oil found in your skin) and thus is highly penetrating and compatible. You can use sunflower or almond oil instead, but be aware that they have a much shorter shelf life.

Don't be alarmed by the quantity of essential oils called for in these recipes, as this is normal for these types of formulations. Because my natural perfume oils are meant to be dabbed onto pulse points, not spritzed over large areas of the body, they are highly aromatic and very safe when used in this manner.

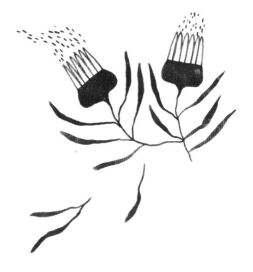

Blue Velvet PERFUME OIL

This is a concentrated version of my adored Blue Velvet Massage Oil (see the recipe on page 71) and is meant to be worn as a sweetly scented yet rich, sultry, woody, and spicy perfume. It definitely leaves an intriguing, lasting impression on all who catch a whiff as you pass by. It appeals to both men and women.

INGREDIENTS

- 12 drops Australian sandalwood essential oil
- 9 drops vanilla (CO₂) essential oil
- 7 drops grapefruit essential oil
- 7 drops juniper berry essential oil
- 5 drops nutmeg essential oil
- 200 IU vitamin E oil
- 2½ teaspoons jojoba oil (or sunflower or almond oil)

Makes about 1 tablespoon

✳ To Make

Combine the sandalwood, vanilla, grapefruit, juniper berry, and nutmeg essential oils in a ½-ounce dark glass bottle with a dropper top or a roller-ball perfume applicator. Add the vitamin E oil, then carefully pour in the jojoba oil. Screw the top on the bottle and shake vigorously for 2 minutes to blend. Label the bottle and store in a dark location at room temperature (between 60° and 80°F) for 2 weeks so the oils can synergize and the fragrance mature. Shake the bottle daily.

Store at room temperature, away from heat and light; use within 2 years (or within 1 year if you used sunflower or almond oil as the base).

✳ To Use

Apply a drop of the perfume oil to several pulse points — inside the wrists and elbows, behind the earlobes, on the temples, at the nape of the neck, under the arms, on cleavage/sternum, behind the knees, on the ankles — up to twice daily.

"Love Is in the Air"
LAVENDER-VETIVER PERFUME OIL

This is a concentrated version of the massage oil on page 67, a seductive scent that's earthy, smoky, warm with light grassy-floral undertones. It's a "lust-have" fragrance for both gals and guys, with calming, grounding, and centering properties. It mellows on the skin, blossoming into an oh-so-sultry aroma.

INGREDIENTS

- 18 drops lavender essential oil
- 12 drops vetiver essential oil
- 200 IU vitamin E oil
- 2½ teaspoons jojoba oil (or sunflower or almond oil)

Makes about 1 tablespoon

✳ To Make

Combine the lavender and vetiver essential oils in a ½-ounce dark glass bottle with a dropper top or a roller-ball perfume applicator. Add the vitamin E oil, then carefully pour in the jojoba oil. Screw the top on the bottle and shake vigorously for 2 minutes to blend. Label the bottle and store in a dark location at room temperature (between 60° and 80°F) for 2 weeks so the oils can synergize and the fragrance mature. Shake the bottle daily.

Store at room temperature, away from heat and light; use within 2 years (or within 1 year if you used sunflower or almond oil as the base).

✳ To Use

Apply a drop to several pulse points — inside the wrists and elbows, behind the earlobes, on the temples, at the nape of the neck, on the cleavage/sternum, under the arms, behind the knees, on the ankles — up to twice daily.

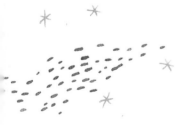

Scentual Treasures to Entice and Delight

AMBER OIL

With its warm, exotic, woody-earthy, and sensual aroma, amber oil is highly prized as a perfume fragrance and is enjoyed equally by both sexes. However, there is no true "amber essential oil," as it's sometimes marketed. Rather, amber oil is an extract of various tree resins, generally found in a solid or semisolid form. For perfume, amber oil is combined with essential oils such as patchouli, sandalwood, styrax, vetiver, cedarwood, davana, and agarwood, plus extracts of frankincense and vanilla, and mixed in a carrier oil. There are many formulations; some have been kept secret for generations by the families that make and sell the fragrant oil blend.

Amber oil is regarded by many as an aphrodisiac, and it's also reputed to promote spiritual enhancement and support meditation because of its grounding properties. Once applied to the skin, it will linger on the body for hours. So, if you enjoy warm, provocative, intoxicating scents and don't mind people asking, "Just what *are* you wearing?" then amber oil may be just the thing!

Be aware that there are many "amber oils" on the market, and quite a few are made with synthetic fragrance oils, so question the retailer (and read the label if possible) before you buy, and purchase only a premium, 100 percent natural blend.

Classic English Lavender
PERFUME OIL #1

A centuries-old classic, this gentle fragrance is an inviting blend of grassy, sweet, herbaceous-floral notes with undertones of balsam and spice. Most people find it appealingly both masculine and feminine; it is one of my absolute favorites.

INGREDIENTS

- 16 drops lavender essential oil
- 8 drops bay laurel essential oil
- 4 drops rosemary essential oil
- 3 drops bergamot essential oil
- 3 drops black pepper essential oil
- 3 drops geranium essential oil
- 200 IU vitamin E oil
- 2½ teaspoons jojoba oil (or sunflower or almond oil)

Makes about 1 tablespoon

✳ To Make

Combine the lavender, bay laurel, rosemary, bergamot, black pepper, and geranium essential oils in a ½-ounce dark glass bottle with a dropper top or a roller-ball perfume applicator. Add the vitamin E oil, then carefully pour in the jojoba oil. Screw the top on the bottle and shake vigorously for 2 minutes to blend. Label the bottle and store in a dark location at room temperature (between 60° and 80°F) for 2 weeks so the oils can synergize and the fragrance mature. Shake the bottle daily.

Store at room temperature, away from heat and light; use within 2 years (or within 1 year if you used sunflower or almond oil as the base).

✳ To Use

Apply a drop to several pulse points — inside the wrists and elbows, behind the earlobes, on the temples, at the nape of the neck, on the cleavage/sternum, under the arms, behind the knees, on the ankles — up to twice daily.

Classic English Lavender
PERFUME OIL #2

Here's another version of the classic English fragrance, but with haunting, soft undertones of musky, herbaceous clary sage and woody cedar. It's not as sweet and green as #1 on the facing page, but it's equally as scentual.

INGREDIENTS

- 19 drops lavender essential oil
- 5 drops clary sage essential oil
- 4 drops cedarwood essential oil
- 3 drops bay laurel essential oil
- 3 drops bergamot essential oil
- 2 drops rosemary essential oil
- 1 drop geranium essential oil
- 200 IU vitamin E oil
- 2½ teaspoons jojoba oil (or sunflower or almond oil)

Makes about 1 tablespoon

✳ To Make

Combine the lavender, clary sage, cedarwood, bay laurel, bergamot, rosemary, and geranium essential oils in a ½-ounce dark glass bottle with a dropper top or a roller-ball perfume applicator. Add the vitamin E oil, then carefully pour in the jojoba oil. Screw the top on the bottle and shake vigorously for 2 minutes to blend. Label the bottle and store in a dark location at room temperature (between 60° and 80°F) for 2 weeks so the oils can synergize and the fragrance mature. Shake the bottle daily.

Store at room temperature, away from heat and light; use within 2 years (or within 1 year if you used sunflower or almond oil as the base).

✳ To Use

Apply a drop to several pulse points — inside the wrists and elbows, behind the earlobes, on the temples, at the nape of the neck, on the cleavage/sternum, under the arms, behind the knees, on the ankles — up to twice daily.

INSTANT Allure

One of the easiest, most convenient ways to scent your body is to apply one drop of essential oil "neat" (undiluted) directly to each of several pulse points, such as inside your wrists and elbows, behind your earlobes, on your temples, at the nape of your neck, under your arms, on your cleavage/sternum, behind your knees, or on your ankles. People who are fond of earthy, sultry sandalwood or patchouli, for instance, often use the pure essential oil as their signature scent.

The vast majority of essential oils must be diluted with a base oil prior to application because of their concentrated nature, but I've found that the pleasingly fragrant essential oils listed below can be tolerated in their undiluted form by many people with nary a problem. If in doubt, perform a patch test to check for skin sensitivity: Just apply a drop of your chosen essential oil to the inside of your elbow and wait a few hours. If you don't react negatively, feel free to apply a few more drops to other pulse points, with a maximum of four drops per day. Avoid contact with your eyes and mucous membranes.

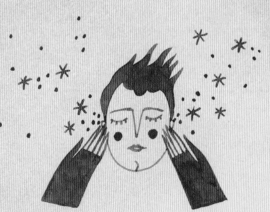

ESSENTIAL OILS TO APPLY NEAT

Lighter Scents

* Geranium

* Lavender

* Neroli

* Petitgrain

Heavier, Richer Scents

* Australian sandalwood

* Cardamom

* Cedarwood

* Frankincense (CO_2)

* Jasmine absolute

* Myrrh

* Patchouli

* Rose absolute

* Vanilla (CO_2)

* Vetiver

* Ylang-ylang

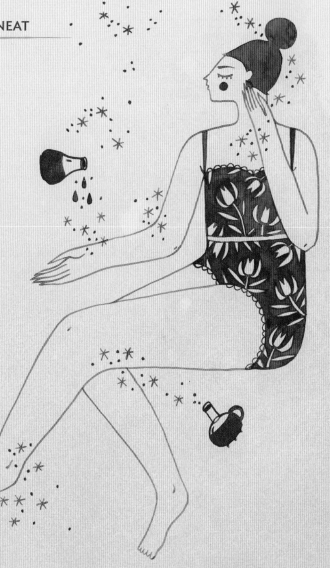

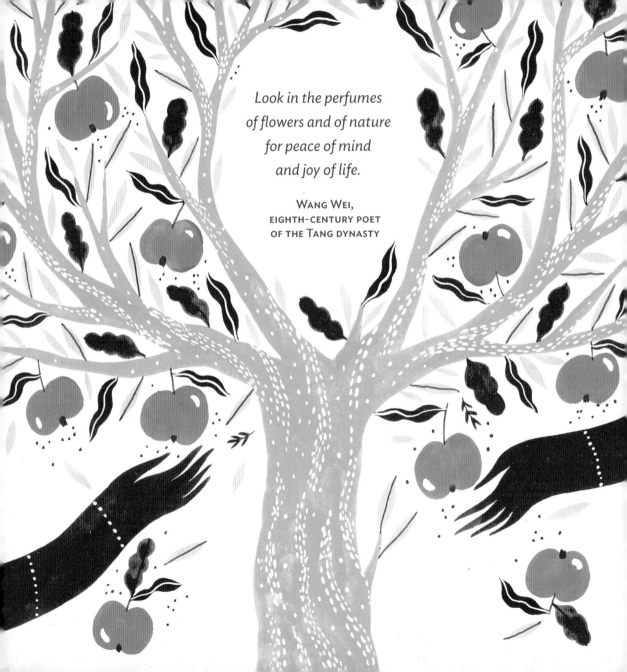

Look in the perfumes
of flowers and of nature
for peace of mind
and joy of life.

WANG WEI,
EIGHTH-CENTURY POET
OF THE TANG DYNASTY

Alluring Solid Perfumes

Solid perfumes are a convenient, unspillable way to carry your scent with you. Since they are oil and wax based, these biocompatible, moisturizing formulations penetrate quickly into warm skin, where they develop and bloom throughout the day, becoming uniquely yours. They're one of my favorite forms of fragrance.

As I noted for perfume oils, you shouldn't be alarmed by the quantity of essential oils called for in the recipes; this is typical for natural perfumes that are to be dabbed onto pulse points and not spritzed over large areas of the body. They are safe when used as directed.

Measuring Beeswax

My solid perfumes use beeswax as a thickener; it's what allows them to be solid. But beeswax brings its own benefits: it's emollient, humectant, skin-conditioning, and antimicrobial. To measure out beeswax, you don't need to grate it (that tends to lead to bloody knuckles). Instead, if you have solid chunks, simply place them in a ziplock freezer bag, and pound them with a hammer into small, measurable pieces. Don't forget that you can always use beeswax pastilles or pellets, as their tiny size makes for convenient and quick measuring. And know that, in general, ½ ounce of beeswax equals 1 tablespoon.

Ruby-Red Rose Solid Perfumes: THREE BLENDS

Sacred to Venus, the Roman goddess of love and sensuality, and intimately connected to her son, Cupid, roses are the universal, fragrant symbol of love, romance, and femininity. If you adore their beauty and exquisite, intoxicating aroma, then you'll favor at least one of these perfume offerings.

INGREDIENTS

- 2 tablespoons plus 1 teaspoon alkanet-infused oil (see recipe, page 44)
- 1 tablespoon beeswax
  Essential oil blend of your choice (see the options on the facing page)

Makes about ¼ cup

To Make

Combine the alkanet oil and beeswax in a very small saucepan or double boiler, and warm over low heat until the beeswax is just melted. Remove from the heat and let cool slightly, for 2 to 3 minutes, stirring a few times to blend. Add the essential oils from your blend of choice and stir again to thoroughly incorporate. Slowly pour the liquid perfume into a 2-ounce jar or tin.

Cap and label, then set aside for 24 hours to allow the essential oils to synergize, the fragrance to develop, and the product to solidify. For maximum aroma and freshness, use within 6 to 12 months.

To Use

Apply a tiny dab to pulse points — inside the wrists and elbows, behind the earlobes, on the temples, at the nape of the neck, on the cleavage/sternum, under the arms, behind the knees, on the ankles — up to twice daily.

CHOOSE YOUR FAVORITE

I offer here three rose-scented essential oil blends from which you can choose as the fragrance for your perfume. A few of the essential oils used in the blends, such as rose absolute, sandalwood, vanilla, and frankincense, are a bit on the expensive side, I'll admit, but consider them an indulgent investment toward enhancing your aromatic aura and sensuality.

Maiden's Blush

A light, soft, rosy floral with herbaceous, slightly sweet notes. Playful, fresh, innocent, yet enticing.

INGREDIENTS

75 drops lavender essential oil
50 drops geranium essential oil
25 drops rose absolute essential oil
20 drops bergamot essential oil
 5 drops vanilla (CO_2) essential oil

New Dawn

A round, rosy-vanilla scent with hints of spicy-green-citrus in the background. An unusual aphrodisiacal blend.

INGREDIENTS

50 drops lemon essential oil
50 drops rose absolute essential oil
30 drops geranium essential oil
30 drops petitgrain essential oil
25 drops Peru balsam essential oil
10 drops frankincense (CO_2) essential oil

Persian Passion

A deeply rich, woody, resinous, spicy blend. The lighter essence of rose floats and dances in the background. Evocative of a sultry, intimately pleasurable evening. Must be experienced; lingers for hours.

INGREDIENTS

40 drops rose absolute essential oil
35 drops Australian sandalwood essential oil
35 drops frankincense (CO_2) essential oil
15 drops patchouli essential oil
 8 drops cinnamon bark essential oil

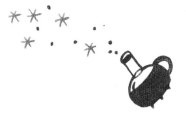

Ravishing Red
ALKANET-INFUSED OIL

Alkanet root is used in the herbal world as a natural red coloring agent for soaps, lip balms, and solid perfumes. It is only soluble in oil, not water.

INGREDIENTS

1 cup sunflower or almond oil (or your favorite neutral oil)

4 tablespoons crushed, dried alkanet root

1,000 IU vitamin E oil

Makes about ¾ cup of oil

✳ To Make

Combine the oil and alkanet root in a pint-size canning jar; cover the mouth of the jar with a piece of plastic wrap and screw on the lid. Shake the mixture for 1 minute. Set the jar in a warm, sunny location, and allow the herb to infuse for 48 hours. Shake the jar twice daily for 30 seconds or so.

Strain the oil through a fine-mesh strainer lined with a fine filter such as muslin or, preferably, a paper coffee filter. Press or squeeze the root bits to extract as much of the precious oil as possible. Strain again if necessary to remove all the particulate matter. Add the vitamin E oil and stir to blend. Pour the oil into a glass storage bottle; label and date. Store at room temperature, away from heat and light; use within 1 year.

✳ To Use

This stunningly beautiful red-hued oil can be used as the base oil for my rose-scented solid perfumes (see page 42). It can also be used as a base oil in my lip balm recipes (see page 86). It will lend a lovely red tint to the finished product but will not deeply stain the lips.

Caution: Alkanet-infused oil will stain light-colored fabrics, so handle with care, and wash your hands after working with it.

SEDUCING THE SENSES

We are inherently sensual beings, and there is no more powerful aphrodisiac than stimulation of our sensual nature. Scent, touch, sound, luscious flavors — when you seduce our senses, you awaken our desire. To entice, titillate, and excite the senses, we use alluring perfumes and colognes, fragrant body oils, scented candles, gentle massage, soulful music, and delectable foods, among other things, in our romantic encounters.

The power of this seduction is clearly evident in the magnitude and longevity of the response it provokes. "Sense memory" is a fairly common, and powerful, experience. Have you ever had a lover who took the time to give you regular massages with a particular aromatic body oil? Does the scent of that oil make you feel relaxed and well loved?

Have you and your beloved ever had a special song? Does it pull at your heartstrings whenever you hear it?

Have you ever had a new lover lie beside you and feed you strawberries, one by one, on a night that ended in a whirlwind of passion? Does your heart skip a beat whenever you see or even smell those luscious berries?

Seduction of the senses is key to arousal and a joyful experience of love — and it builds up to a long, reverberating resonance in the soul. In fact, the aphrodisiac effect of many "love potions" lies in their appeal to the senses. So give yourself over to absolute sensual pleasure. Don't feel guilty — explore it, embrace it, experience it. Healthy loving is part of healthy living. Never forget that!

AROMATIC TRESSES

No matter whether you're a man or a woman, being known for having hair that smells wonderful can be part of your signature "fragrance style." So if you want to stand out in a crowd, or if you think your partner could use a bit of a pleasant surprise, consider imbuing your hair with the enthralling natural aromas of essential oils and hydrosols.

Aromatic hydrosols such as rose, rose geranium, lemon verbena, neroli, peppermint, rosemary, and cucumber are good choices. You spritz them on damp or dry hair any time of day.

Essential oils that can be applied neat (undiluted), such as Australian sandalwood, myrrh, frankincense (CO_2), geranium, rose, lavender, cardamom, neroli, jasmine, vanilla (CO_2), Roman chamomile, cedarwood, lavender, and rosemary verbenon, can be distributed through your hair simply by working a couple of drops through damp or dry hair with your hands. Or put a couple of drops on your hairbrush before using it. Just be careful not to get essential oils in your eyes, nose, or mouth.

If you love the rich, creamy, sweet scent of vanilla beans, apply a few drops of premium Madagascar vanilla extract to your tresses, especially to the hair at the nape of your neck, where it will mingle with the warmth of your skin and blossom into your own unique fragrance. It's absolutely exquisite!

Sea Salt Seduction

SOLID PERFUME

This unisex blend of citrus, spice, and resin yields a seductive fragrance that starts on a fresh note of citrus peel and mellows into an aroma reminiscent of warm sands and ocean breezes, with a hint of natural musk. This scent will take you there.

INGREDIENTS

- 2 tablespoons plus 1 teaspoon sunflower or almond oil
- 1 tablespoon beeswax
- 95 drops lime essential oil
- 30 drops ginger essential oil
- 30 drops grapefruit essential oil
- 20 drops petitgrain essential oil
- 10 drops bergamot essential oil
- 10 drops black pepper essential oil
- 5 drops frankincense (CO_2) essential oil

Makes about ¼ cup

✳ To Make

Combine the sunflower oil and beeswax in a very small saucepan or double boiler, and warm over low heat until the beeswax is just melted. Remove from the heat and let cool slightly, for 2 to 3 minutes, stirring a few times to blend. Add the essential oils and stir again to thoroughly incorporate. Slowly pour the liquid perfume into a 2-ounce jar or tin. Cap and label, then set aside for 24 hours to allow the essential oils to synergize, the fragrance to develop, and the product to reach a solid consistency. Because of the large percentage of highly volatile citrus oils, use within 6 months for maximum aroma and freshness.

✳ To Use

Apply a tiny dab to pulse points — inside the wrists and elbows, behind the earlobes, on the temples, at the nape of the neck, under the arms, on the cleavage/sternum, behind the knees, under the arms, on the ankles — up to twice daily.

Caution: Because of the high concentration of citrus oils, this perfume may cause skin irritation or photosensitivity. Avoid application to skin that will be exposed to the sun.

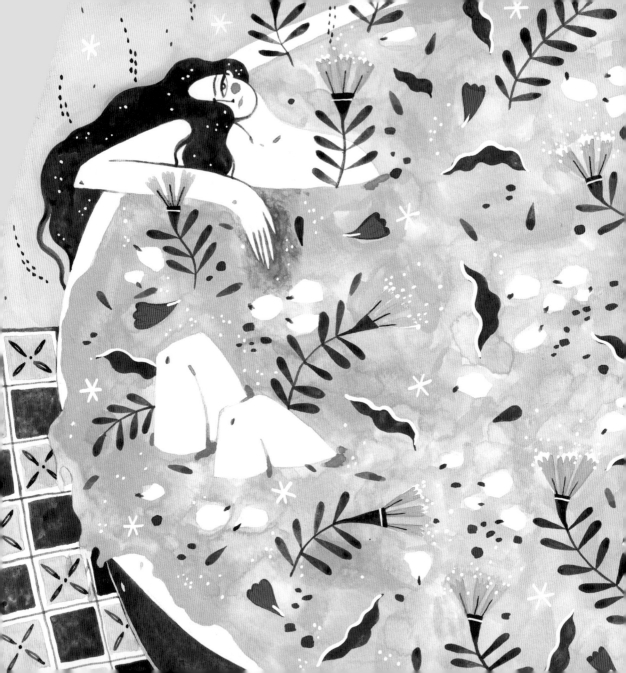

CHAPTER 3

Aromatic Baths
to Silken the Skin and Set the Mood

BATHING ENJOYS A RICH and redolent history. Cleopatra was known for taking soothing, skin-lightening baths in fresh ass's milk; Marie Antoinette reputedly enjoyed long, luxurious herbal soaks; and the women of the ancient Arabian harems were renowned for their satiny skin, luminous complexions, and bathing rituals that often lasted for hours and included exfoliating with fine granular pastes consisting of oil-rich seeds and spices, anointing their bodies with perfumed oils, and enjoying soothing massages. The ancient Greek and Roman public baths — elaborate, ornate structures, often constructed of marble — provided individuals of all classes the opportunity to cleanse themselves, exercise, and unwind, while also serving as gathering places for the community to both socialize and conduct business.

Unfortunately, the pace of modern living has caused the shower to replace the bath in popularity, but let me be clear: showering is fine for a quick cleanup, but it is no replacement for a long, luxurious soak. Bathing is a wonderful way to pamper and soothe yourself, rejuvenate, relax, and refresh the senses. It is a tactile aphrodisiac, honoring the sense of touch and opening the way to intimacy.

A bath can also create some much-needed private time to bask in skin-conditioning water infused with the natural goodness of fragrant oils, herbs, salts, and bubbles. It's vitally important for us to take time out to create a space of tranquility in which to nurture ourselves. Then we can pass along that peacefulness to others — especially to our sweeties.

With the right ingredients, a bath can be a therapeutic treatment for the mind, body, and spirit: 30 minutes after stepping into the bath you can emerge a new person, having left behind the frustrations and worries of the day. Your skin will be delicately scented, soft and silky to the touch, leaving you feeling ever-so-loving and beautiful, prepared for an evening of intimacy with your beloved.

Note: Please keep bathwater warm, not hot. The hotter the water, the quicker the volatile essential oils (if you're using them) dissipate into the air and lose their healing qualities. And hot water dehydrates your skin.

Coconut Milk Bath

Did you know that canned, full-fat coconut milk can be added to the bath as a highly moisturizing, deliciously scented skin softener? For skin that smells incredibly edible and whispers, "Touch me," simply pour half of a 14-ounce can directly under the running bathwater (save the other half for another bath or add it to your daily smoothie). The coconut oil floats, and the mineral-rich milk disperses. Step in, relax, and luxuriate for about 20 minutes. Prior to drying off, take a few minutes to massage the tropical oil into your skin.

NATURAL BODY ODOR
Turn-On or Turn-Off?

As a general rule, a healthy body produces a healthy odor, ranging from almost undetectable to moderately strong but inoffensive. Natural human scent, unmasked by deodorants or overly scented soap, can be a powerful attraction factor and arousal stimulant. Some people actually prefer the natural, slightly musky aroma of their partner that develops within several hours to a day after a bath rather than their just-washed, scentless body. Legend has it that whenever Napoleon was traveling back to his beloved Josephine, he sent a messenger ahead to instruct her not to bathe for three days prior to his arrival, as he much adored her lovely unwashed essence.

Scent preference is an individual thing, and every person has a unique scent signature. As an experiment, try forgoing commercial deodorant and deodorizing soap for a week; instead use a natural, essential oil–based liquid deodorant or body powder and pure olive oil or herb-infused natural soap. These will gently minimize body odor but allow some of your personal essence to develop. See what your partner has to say about your new scent — perhaps it will lead to an interesting evening!

Honey Cream BATH

An ultra-pampering, luxurious bath blend formulated to moisturize and hydrate the driest of skin. The combination of emollient cream with soothing, healing, humectant honey will leave your skin feeling silky and kissably soft, with a lingering, light aromatic essence of sweet honey.

INGREDIENTS

- 1 cup heavy cream or half-and-half, preferably organic
- ½ cup raw honey

✳ To Make

Pour the cream and the honey together directly under running bathwater. Swish the water with your hands to mix before getting into the tub.

✳ To Use

Relax. Submerge your entire body for about 20 minutes. Pat dry, and follow with an application of your favorite moisturizer, if desired.

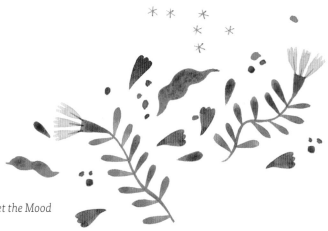

Soft-as-Silk
AROMATHERAPEUTIC MILK BATH

For skin that's deeply moisturized and touchably soft, this simple yet indulgent milk bath is sure to please. Customize it by choosing an essential oil that benefits your emotional and physical needs.

INGREDIENTS

- ¾ cup powdered milk (whole or nonfat), preferably organic
- 1 tablespoon jojoba, sunflower, almond, or your favorite oil
- 8 drops essential oil(s) of your choice (see the list at right)

✳ To Make

Pour the powdered milk and oil together directly under the running bathwater. When the tub is full, add the essential oil, then step into the tub. Swish the water with your hands to mix.

✳ To Use

Relax. Submerge your entire body in this moisturizing bath for about 20 minutes. Pat dry, and follow with an application of your favorite moisturizer, if desired.

Milk Bath Essential Oils

Calming & soothing

Lavender, patchouli, vetiver, Roman chamomile, Australian sandalwood, vanilla (CO_2)

Stimulating

Ginger, cardamom, allspice, cedarwood

Gently uplifting & balancing

Geranium, petitgrain, rose, palmarosa, frankincense

Garden of Flowers
RELAXING BATH

This bath blend was created for the flower gardener in all of us. I chose calendula especially for its skin-rejuvenating and healing properties, chamomile and lavender for their ability to ease tense nerves and tight muscles, and roses, well, simply for their sublime scent. There's nothing quite like steeping yourself in a tub of fragrant herb tea infused with milky oats — it's a most sensuous experience, soothing to the psyche as well as the flesh.

INGREDIENTS

- ½ cup instant or old-fashioned oats
- 2 tablespoons dried or 4 tablespoons fresh calendula petals
- 2 tablespoons dried or 4 tablespoons fresh chamomile flowers
- 2 tablespoons dried or 4 tablespoons fresh lavender buds
- 2 tablespoons dried or 4 tablespoons fresh rose petals
- 5 drops geranium essential oil
- 5 drops lavender essential oil

✳ To Make

Combine the oats, calendula petals, chamomile flowers, lavender buds, and rose petals in a muslin bag, handkerchief, or square of double-thick cheesecloth. Add the geranium and lavender essential oils and tie up tightly. Hang from the nozzle of the tub. Turn on the tap and let the water pour through the bath bag. When the tub is full, untie the bag and let it float in the water.

✳ To Use

Step in and relax. Submerge your entire body for about 20 minutes. As you soak, gently rub your body with the bag, using it as an herbal washcloth. Pat dry, and follow with an application of your favorite moisturizer, if desired.

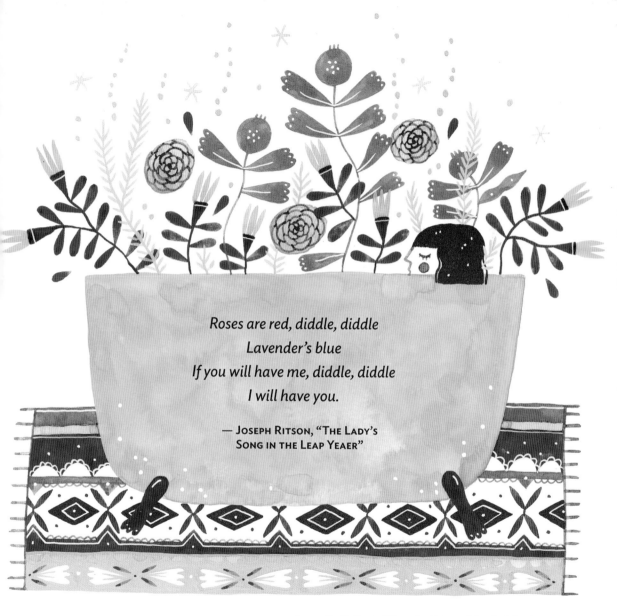

Roses are red, diddle, diddle
Lavender's blue
If you will have me, diddle, diddle
I will have you.

— JOSEPH RITSON, "THE LADY'S
SONG IN THE LEAP YEAER"

Cinnamon, Ginger & Orange
STIMULATING BATH SALTS

This stimulating, warming, slightly spicy "feel good" bath blend helps relieve lethargy and muscle aches while simultaneously softening and scenting the skin with a fragrance that appeals to both men and women.

INGREDIENTS

- ½ cup baking soda
- ½ cup sea salt
- 1 tablespoon ground cinnamon
- 1 tablespoon ground ginger
- 1 tablespoon dried (or 2 tablespoons fresh) finely chopped orange peel
- 2 teaspoons jojoba, sunflower, almond, or your favorite oil
- 3 drops ginger essential oil (optional)
- 3 drops sweet orange essential oil (optional)

✳ To Make

Combine the baking soda, sea salt, cinnamon, ginger, and orange peel in a muslin bag, handkerchief, or square of double-thick cheesecloth. Add the base oil and essential oils, if desired, to the mix, and tie up tightly. Hang from the nozzle of the tub. Turn on the tap and let the water pour through the bath bag, turning your tub into a salty, soothing infusion of spices and oils. When the tub is full, untie the bag and let it float in the water.

✳ To Use

Step in and relax. Soak for about 20 minutes. Pat dry, and follow with an application of your favorite moisturizer, if desired.

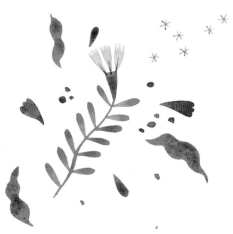

Essence of Roses
MILKY BATH SALTS

Indulgent, to say the least, this blend of skin-silkening powdered milk and muscle-relaxing, mineral-rich sea salt combined with intoxicatingly fragrant rose petals will surely pamper your body and put you in the mood for love.

INGREDIENTS

- ¾ cup powdered milk (whole or nonfat), preferably organic
- ¾ cup sea salt
- 1 cup dried or 2 cups fresh rose petals, preferably organic
- 10 drops essential oil(s) of your choice

To Make

Combine the powdered milk, sea salt, and rose petals in a muslin bag, handkerchief, or square of double-thick cheesecloth. Add the essential oil to the mix and tie up tightly. Hang from the nozzle of the tub. Turn on the tap and let the water pour through the bath bag, turning your tub into a delectable, soothing infusion of skin-softening luxury. When the tub is full, untie the bag and let it float in the water.

To Use

Step in and submerge yourself for about 20 minutes. As you soak, gently rub your entire body with the bag, using it as a rose-scented washcloth. Pat dry, and follow with an application of your favorite moisturizer, if desired.

NOTE: For the essential oils I like a blend of palmarosa, geranium, and rose absolute, but you can customize the rosy scent to your liking — just don't use more than 10 drops total.

BATH OILS
Nourishing Luxury for Your Skin

Food-grade, unrefined, minimally processed, and preferably organic nut, seed, bean, and fruit oils act as nutrient-rich lubricants and emollient moisture barriers; they help keep your skin elastic, soft, and hydrated following a bath. Simply add 1 tablespoon of oil to the bathtub as you fill it. Step in, relax and soak for about 20 minutes, and luxuriate in the skin-pampering goodness. Pat dry. Your skin should feel invitingly soft and sensuous!

My favorite bath oil is jojoba, as it does not need refrigeration, will not go rancid, is chemically similar to human sebum, and penetrates quite readily, but slightly lighter oils such as apricot kernel, almond, sunflower, and soybean also work well (though they must be refrigerated). Sesame, avocado, and extra-virgin olive oil are heavy and can have a quite distinctive aroma that you may dislike — though sesame oil or real, raw, pure olive oil can impart an incredibly velvety texture to the skin that I love, especially in midwinter, when my skin is driest. Extra-virgin coconut oil is a favored bath oil for many who enjoy the exquisite tropical fragrance.

If you prefer fragrant bath oils, all of my massage oil recipes in the following chapter double as wonderful bath oils.

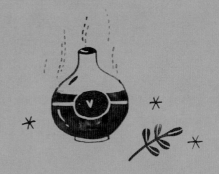

Bubblicious Herbal
BATH FOAM

There's something playful, magical, and sensuous about submerging yourself in a tub full of fluffy, fragrant bubbles. This recipe is an easy-to-make alternative to chemical-laden commercial foaming bath products. A multipurpose formulation, it can also be used as a hair shampoo, body wash, or liquid hand soap, and it makes a great travel cleanser! Note that natural foaming agents do not produce quite as many billowy suds as commercial products.

INGREDIENTS

40 drops essential oils
1 (8-ounce) bottle natural shampoo, unscented

Makes 1 cup

✳ To Make

Add the essential oil(s) to the bottle of shampoo and shake well to blend.

✳ To Use

Turn on the tap full blast and squirt 2 to 4 tablespoons of the bath foam into the tub. Step in and relax, submerging your entire body in bubbles for about 20 minutes. Pat dry, and follow with an application of your favorite moisturizer, if desired.

NOTE: For the essential oils, consider lavender, rosemary verbenon, spearmint, geranium, palmarosa, vanilla (CO_2), ylang-ylang, patchouli, Australian sandalwood, cardamom, rose absolute, frankincense (CO_2), or myrrh.

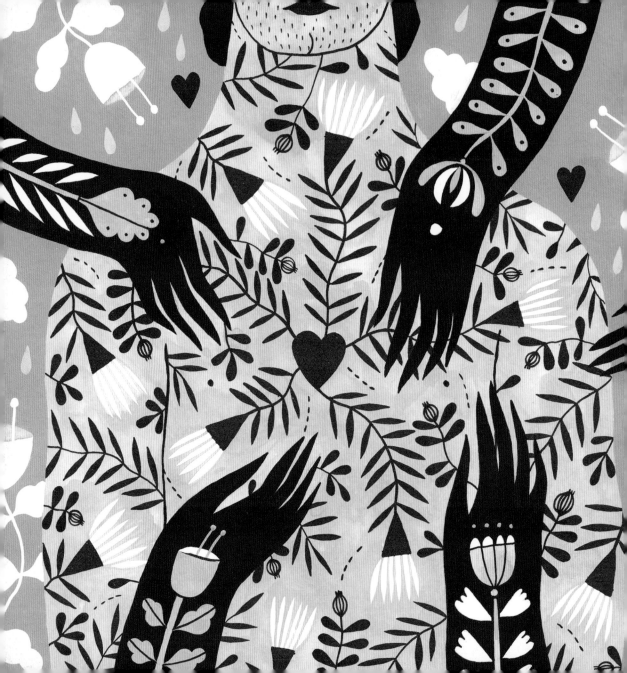

CHAPTER 4

Luxurious Oils
for Sensual Massage

TOUCH IS THE OLDEST AND TRUEST form of communion, and far as I'm concerned, there's no better way of showing your beloved that you deeply care for his or her well-being than by giving a loving, soothing massage. Whether it's undertaken with the intent of pure relaxation or as titillating foreplay, or it's therapeutic or exquisitely sensual, massage is a celebration of physical intimacy, a wonderful way of allowing your loving energy to flow through your hands into your partner, encouraging slow, deep destressing and opening of the heart.

In today's fast-paced world of expensive and technological gadgetry, futilely designed to increase the physical enjoyment of life, it is enormously satisfying to realize that you can give — and simultaneously receive — so much happiness and pleasure by just using your two hands. Think about it: Happiness and pleasure are two of life's most potent medicines, sending the right stimuli to the body's cells to keep them healthy. Massage helps the nerves to relax while at the same time stimulating the senses. It may just be the perfect aphrodisiac!

Giving a Good
Full-Body Massage

Many excellent books exist with detailed instructions in the art of massage, and I'd encourage you to expand your knowledge a bit by further study. A couple of my oldie-but-goodie favorites are listed in the recommended reading section (page 168). If you've had some basic training in massage therapy, that's great, but it's not vital, as long as you observe some simple principles:

* **DIM THE LIGHTS.** Make it easy for your partner to totally relax and drift off if he or she wishes. Lighting should be soft and indirect. Candlelight sets a romantic mood, as does working in darkness with the full moon streaming in through the windows.

* **TRIM YOUR FINGERNAILS.** Your hands should be as soft and smooth as possible, and this includes having fingernails that are filed neatly and trimmed short enough so as not to scratch your partner's skin.

* **SUGGEST A WARMING BATH.** Your partner may want to take a shower or warm bath before the massage. Warm water relaxes and softens muscle tissue, making the massage even more pleasurable for your partner and easier on your hands, as well.

* **WARMTH IS ESSENTIAL,** for both the room and your hands. You're doing all the work, but your partner barely moves; thus he or she may feel chilled when you're feeling fine or even a bit toasty. Seventy-five degrees is usually comfortable. If

your hands tend to be cold, warm them first by immersing them in very warm water for a couple of minutes — simply rubbing your palms together isn't enough.

* **QUIET, PLEASE.** Turn off your phone. Lock the door. Hang up a DO NOT DISTURB sign. Make sure children and pets have been attended to — this is your special time with no distractions. If you like music, put on something smooth and easy. In an outdoor setting, Mother Nature provides her own soothing sounds.

* **FIND A COMFORTABLE PLATFORM.** Perform massage on a stable, relatively level surface. A bed, a futon cushion, several yoga mats or quilts stacked one atop the other, or a thick rug will work well. Obviously, a massage table works, too. Cover surfaces with soft sheets that you don't mind getting oily or lightly stained. If outdoors, find a level grassy bit of ground or sandy beach, and smooth over any lumps and grit with a heavy blanket.

* **USE SUPPORTIVE PILLOWS.** If possible, place a pillow under your partner's knees while massaging the front of the body, and under his or her ankles and tummy while massaging the back.

* **SCENT YOUR SURROUNDINGS.** Many couples use long-burning incense, an aromatherapy diffuser, or a candle to heighten the experience with sensual fragrance. Be careful, though, not to assault the senses, especially if you're already using an aromatic massage oil.

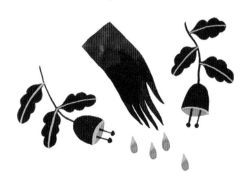

* **BE PREPARED.** Have everything on hand before you start. This includes gently warmed massage oil, a large towel to cover the areas not being worked on, two glasses of water, finger food, a few hand towels for cleanup, a robe for your partner, and so on, so that the sensual atmosphere is not disturbed while you scurry off to find something.

* **USE MASSAGE OIL CORRECTLY.** Never pour or squirt massage oil directly onto your partner as it can be a jolting experience. Rather, pour the oil into your palm and gently rub your hands together so that the oil is evenly dispersed; then apply it to your partner's body. Oiling is a delicious feeling — let your partner relish it!

* **KEEP IN TOUCH.** All massage movements should blend together in a single, smooth, slow motion. Using the full surface of your hands, keep your fingers together. Touch and stroke as much as possible during the entire massage. When you move from one part of the body to another, always keep one hand on your partner's body, making the contact seem continuous and a part of the massage. Repeat movements several times, and if your partner really likes something that you're doing, keep it up for a while longer.

* **PUT YOUR HEART INTO IT.** The act of massage is intimate and beautiful. Put your heart into what you're doing and thoroughly enjoy it. It's beneficial for you as well as your beloved.

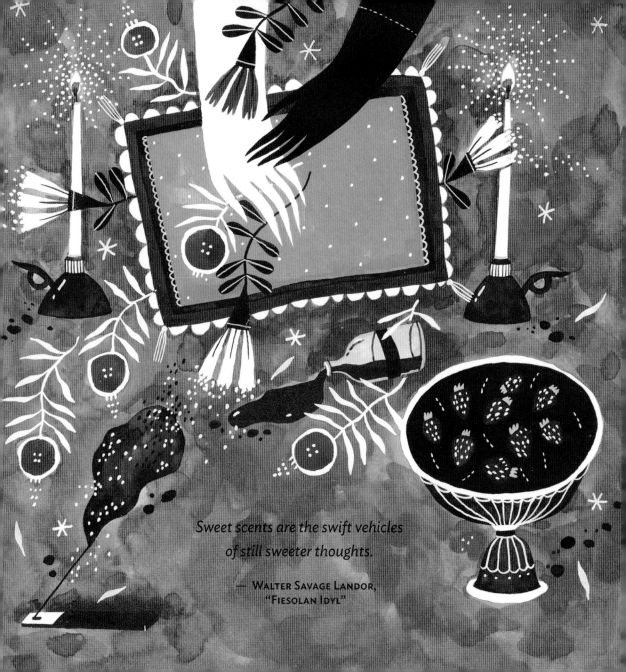

Sweet scents are the swift vehicles
of still sweeter thoughts.

— Walter Savage Landor,
"Fiesolan Idyl"

Massage Oil Blends

My aromatherapeutic oil blends are designed specifically to inspire and enhance the massage experience. So forget about time and schedules, indulge the senses, and enjoy some beautifully blissful touch!

Note: In my opinion, massage oils are best applied to the skin while it's still warm from a shower or bath, when I feel the skin's pores are relaxed, encouraging deep absorption of the skin-nourishing nutrients from the oil and the aromatherapeutic properties of the essential oils you've used. But the natural, unrefined oils called for in my recipes — primarily jojoba, sunflower, almond, coconut, and avocado — penetrate the skin so easily that they can be applied anytime you wish. These wonderful oils leave your skin deeply moisturized, glowing with vitality, and healthy from the inside out.

"Love Is in the Air"
LAVENDER-VETIVER MASSAGE OIL

Provocative vetiver brings the warmth, and lovely lavender brings the sweet, producing an earthy, smoky, exotic aroma with light grassy-floral undertones and a unisex appeal. It mellows on the skin, blossoming into an oh-so-sultry scent. Couples with a high-stress lifestyle will find this aphrodisiacal blend much to their liking, as it delivers calming, grounding, and centering properties while stirring flames of passion. For a more potent scent, try a lavender-vetiver perfume oil; see the recipe on page 34.

INGREDIENTS

36 drops lavender essential oil

28 drops vetiver essential oil

1 cup jojoba oil (or sunflower or almond oil)

1,000 IU vitamin E oil

Makes about 1 cup

✳ To Make

Combine the lavender and vetiver essential oils in an 8-ounce glass or plastic storage bottle. Add the jojoba oil and vitamin E. Screw the top on the bottle and shake vigorously to blend the ingredients. Label the bottle and place in a dark location at room temperature (between 60° and 80°F) for 24 hours so the oils can synergize. Store at room temperature, away from heat and light; use within 2 years (or within 1 year if you used sunflower or almond oil as the base).

✳ To Use

Shake well before each use. Apply whenever you wish, whether for massage or as a deeply penetrating body oil. For use as a bath oil, add 1 tablespoon to running water, step in, and luxuriate in earthly blissfulness!

Vanilla Intrigue
MASSAGE OIL

Soft, warm, delicious, almost intoxicating, with a rich vanilla bean aroma, this scentsational oil is adored by both men and women. It easily melts into the skin, leaving a velvety finish, with no oily residue, and is ideal for use during a massage or as a full-body moisturizing perfume. Simply fabulous!

INGREDIENTS

6 long vanilla beans or 100 drops vanilla (CO_2) essential oil

1½ cups jojoba oil

1,000 IU vitamin E oil

Makes about 1½ cups

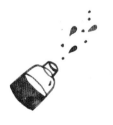

✳ To Make

Slice the vanilla beans lengthwise, scrape out the paste from each pod, and add it to a pint-size glass jar. Chop the empty bean pods into ½-inch pieces and add them to the jar. Pour in the jojoba oil and vitamin E oil. (Add the vanilla essential oil now if you're using it instead of vanilla beans.) Place a piece of plastic wrap over the jar, screw on the lid, and shake the mixture for 1 minute.

Store the jar in a dark place for 2 months (or longer — the longer it steeps, the stronger the scent) to allow the vanilla essence to infuse the oil. During this time shake the jar every day for 10 to 15 seconds.

After 2 months strain the oil through a fine-mesh strainer or a strainer lined with a coffee filter to remove all the particulate matter. The finished oil will have a deep, round vanilla fragrance and pale golden-brown color. Pour the oil into a storage container (an elegant glass bottle is nice, though a plastic squeeze bottle is more convenient for use). Label and date. Store at room temperature, away from heat and light; use within 2 years.

✳ To Use

Shake well before each use. Apply whenever you wish, whether for massage or as a deeply penetrating body oil. For use as a bath oil, add 1 tablespoon to running water, step in, and feel pampered.

Variation: For a warm, sensual, spicy massage oil, add 1 tablespoon cardamom seeds and 4 broken cinnamon sticks along with the vanilla beans.

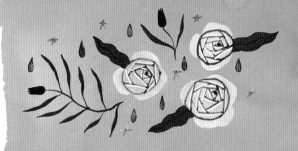

*Yes, it's true
the senses can lead you astray
and the pursuit of pleasure
can get you in trouble.
Sensual pleasure
needs the guidance of practical
and ethical judgment.
But you won't gain good health
by repeatedly vetoing the vote
of the senses and denigrating
the wisdom of the body.
Nature was neither capricious nor
perverted in making sure
that, other things being equal,
what feels good is good for you.*

— GEORGE LEONARD

Warm and Sweet Relaxing
MASSAGE OIL

A caring, relaxing massage at the end of a long day is one of the best ways to enkindle intimacy and closeness with your beloved. This warming blend, with its luscious combination of sweet, spicy, woodsy, apple-like aromas, contains essential oils with properties known to ease tight and tense muscles, calm the nerves, and relieve anxiety — the perfect inducement for an evening of tranquility.

INGREDIENTS

26 drops Roman chamomile essential oil

22 drops sweet marjoram essential oil

16 drops cardamom essential oil

1 cup jojoba oil (or sunflower or almond oil)

1,000 IU vitamin E oil

Makes about 1 cup

✳ To Make

Combine the Roman chamomile, sweet marjoram, and cardamom essential oils in an 8-ounce glass or plastic storage bottle. Add the jojoba oil and vitamin E. Screw the top on the bottle and shake vigorously to blend all the ingredients. Label the bottle and place in a dark location at room temperature (between 60° and 80°F) for 24 hours so the oils can synergize. Store at room temperature, away from heat and light; use within 2 years (or within 1 year if you used sunflower or almond oil as the base).

✳ To Use

Shake well before each use. Apply whenever you wish, whether for massage or as a deeply penetrating body oil. For use as a bath oil, add 1 tablespoon to running water, step in, and unwind.

Blue Velvet
MASSAGE OIL

Ultrasmooth, round, and velvety soft, this blend of woody, spicy, and sweetly scented essential oils, with unisex appeal, is a rich, skin-conditioning, gliding mixture of nourishing, indulgent ingredients with which to massage your beloved and heighten moments of passion. It pampers, silkens, and warms the skin. I often wear it as a scented body oil — absolutely delectable! For a more potent version of this scent, see the recipe for Blue Velvet Perfume Oil (page 33).

INGREDIENTS

- 24 drops Australian sandalwood essential oil
- 18 drops vanilla (CO_2) essential oil
- 14 drops grapefruit essential oil
- 14 drops juniper berry essential oil
- 10 drops nutmeg essential oil
- ½ cup sunflower or almond oil
- ½ cup avocado oil
- 1,000 IU vitamin E oil

Makes about 1 cup

✳ To Make

Combine the sandalwood, vanilla, grapefruit, juniper berry, and nutmeg essential oils in an 8-ounce glass or plastic storage bottle. Add the sunflower oil, avocado oil, and vitamin E. Screw the top on the bottle and shake vigorously to blend all the ingredients. Label the bottle and place in a dark location at room temperature (between 60° and 80°F) for 24 hours so the oils can synergize. Store at room temperature, away from heat and light; use within 1 year.

✳ To Use

Shake well before each use. Apply whenever you wish, whether for massage or as a deeply penetrating body oil. For use as a bath oil, add 1 tablespoon to running water, step in, and feel spoiled. You deserve it!

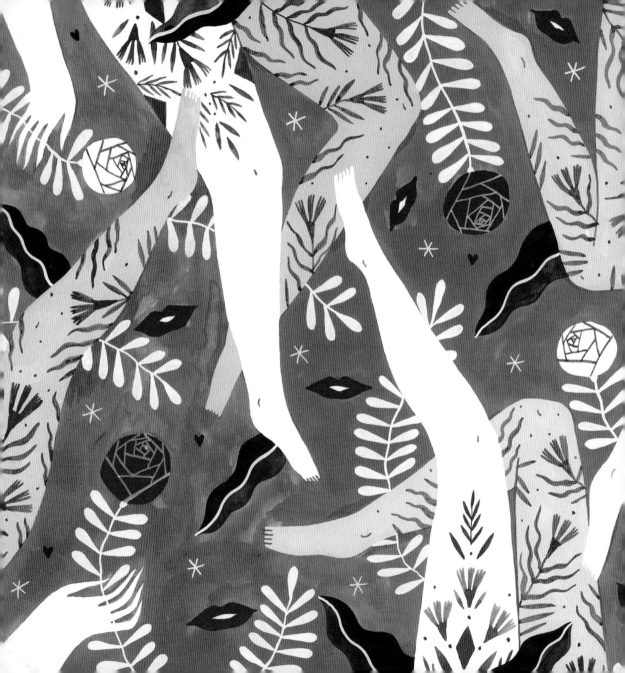

CHAPTER 5

Edible Body Butters, Balms & Lubricants

CREATED ESPECIALLY FOR YOU and your lover to share and delight in, these sweet, spicy, savory, and bawdy body treats add delicious flavor and fun to your lovemaking rituals. Experience some tasty pleasure, invigorate the senses, make the ordinary extraordinary — let your imagination run wild! Frolic and play with your partner, and spread a yummy coating on any body part you fancy. And enjoy at will — all of these recipes are completely edible and chemical-free.

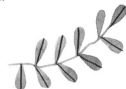

"Sex on the Beach"

COCOA-COCONUT LOVE BUTTER

Evoking the essence of tropical beaches, this buttery blend is oh-so-sensual and inviting. Its three oil-rich ingredients nourish and lubricate the skin — and happily, they're edible. Slather some on, and with your skin feeling so soft and smelling so absolutely scrumptious, your lover might just want to devour you for dinner . . .

INGREDIENTS

- 5 tablespoons unrefined extra-virgin coconut oil
- 2 tablespoons almond or sunflower oil
- 1 tablespoon cocoa butter

Makes about ½ cup

✳ To Make

Combine the coconut oil, almond oil, and cocoa butter in a small saucepan or double boiler and warm over low heat until all the solids are just melted. Remove from the heat and let cool for 5 to 10 minutes, stirring a few times to blend. Pour into a 4-ounce jar or tin, cap, and label. (Since coconut oil is solid below 76°F and liquid at higher temperatures, you may prefer to store the formula in a plastic squeeze bottle in warmer weather.)

Store at room temperature, away from heat and light; use within 1 year. This formula is slow to thicken and may require up to 24 hours to reach its final creamy, buttery texture.

✳ To Use

If the butter is in liquid form, shake well before each use. I believe it is best applied to the skin while it's still warm from a shower or bath. But honestly, it penetrates so easily that you can apply it anytime.

Caution: This butter is not latex-friendly.

Smooth & Sensual

CINNAMON-COCOA LOVE BUTTER

This soothing, aromatic love balm warms and gently tingles on contact. A universal favorite, cinnamon's spicy-sweet taste and fragrance are enjoyed by both men and women, and when it's blended with chocolaty cocoa butter, the result is a "love lube" that suggests, "Come play with me."

INGREDIENTS

- 2 tablespoons plus 1 teaspoon sunflower or almond oil (or your favorite neutral oil)
- 1 tablespoon cocoa butter
- 1 teaspoon vegetable glycerin
- 1 teaspoon beeswax
  Cinnamon flavoring oil

Makes about ¼ cup

NOTE: If you omit the cinnamon flavoring, you can use this balm as a slightly sweet personal lubricant. This skin-conditioning formula doubles as a superior lip balm, cuticle softener, and foot cream.

✳ To Make

Combine the sunflower oil, cocoa butter, glycerin, and beeswax in a very small saucepan or double boiler and warm over low heat until the solids are just melted. Remove from the heat and let cool for a few minutes, stirring a few times to blend. Add the cinnamon flavoring oil to taste, mixing it in 1 drop at a time (a little goes a *long* way). Then steadily beat the mixture with a small spoon for a few minutes until it begins to thicken slightly and become opaque. This ensures that the water-based glycerin is thoroughly incorporated. Pour or spoon into a 2-ounce jar or tin. Cap, label, and set aside for 4 hours to synergize and thicken completely. No refrigeration is required, but for maximum aroma and taste, use within 1 year.

✳ To Use

This formula can be used as a highly emollient, tasty kissing balm, or you can spread it wherever you desire some caressing.

Caution: This butter is not latex-friendly.

BODY GHEE: *Sumptuous & Savory*

Love the rich, savory, fatty taste of butter and the way it slips and slides in your mouth? "Everything's better with butter," as the saying goes, and some couples enjoy using ghee, or clarified butter, as a natural, edible "love lube" and massage oil. Ghee is made by ever-so-slowly cooking pure, unsalted, sweet cream butter to coax out both the water and milk solids (proteins). What remains is a luxurious, semisoft, oily spread with a rich buttery taste and aroma.

Ghee melts upon contact with the body. It's an amazing skin conditioner, and the way it tastes on warm flesh is downright heavenly! It can be scooped right out of the jar and used plain, or you can enhance the flavor by combining a couple of tablespoons of ghee in a small bowl with a few drops of sweet-tasting vegetable glycerin, along with a couple of drops of orange, vanilla, or cardamom essential oil. Spread it anywhere you want, especially in areas that benefit from lubrication, or all over the body as a deeply conditioning, full-body massage oil — it'll leave the skin satiny soft. (But note: ghee is not latex-friendly.)

Bodacious Coconut–Vanilla
BODY DESSERT

Coconut oil and vanilla bean paste — a simple combination that produces an exotic, sweet-tasting, slippery, aromatic sensation that is sure to pleasure and please. While experimenting with this recipe, I found myself eating it by the spoonful. It's that good!

INGREDIENTS

- 3 tablespoons extra-virgin, unrefined coconut oil
- 2–3 teaspoons vanilla bean paste, sweetened with sugar (use the greater amount for more intense flavor and sweetness)

Makes about ¼ cup

✳ To Make

If the coconut oil is hard, set the container in a bowl of hot water for 10 minutes or so until it softens. Place the coconut oil in a very small bowl (a custard cup works great). Add the vanilla paste and rapidly whisk the two together to blend. Scoop into a little pretty jar, and store in the refrigerator, where it will keep for up to 2 months — if it lasts that long!

✳ To Use

This edible body dessert will harden in the fridge, but the coconut oil will melt easily when it's massaged into the skin. Spread it anywhere you want to kiss or be kissed. Your skin will become slightly sticky and very soft.

Caution: This balm is not latex-friendly.

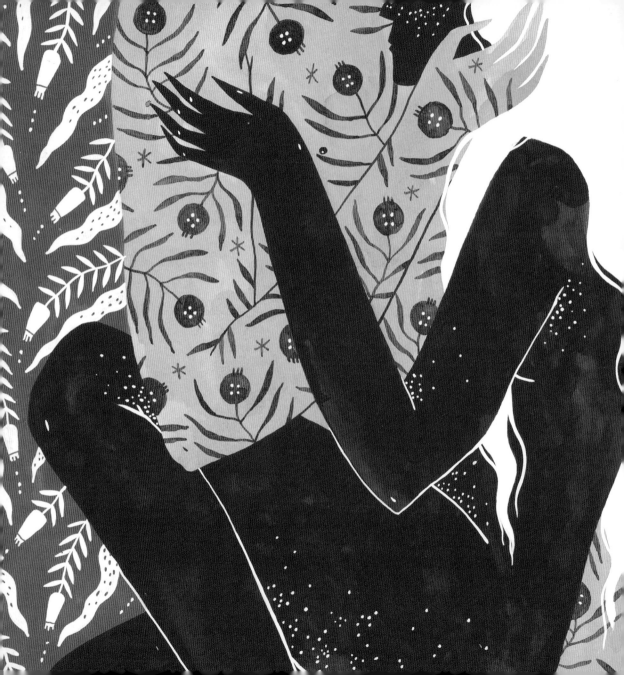

Sweet Pleasure
BODY HONEY

This edible blend is fabulously tasty, aromatic, and easy to make. It's also comforting to dry skin and works wonderfully well as a hydrating sensual lubricant.

INGREDIENTS

- 1 tablespoon extra-virgin, unrefined coconut oil
- ½ teaspoon raw honey
- 1–2 drops vanilla, peppermint, spearmint, fennel, cinnamon bark, or sweet orange essential oil, or your favorite flavoring oil such as almond, hazelnut, cherry, peach, or strawberry

Makes about 1 heaping tablespoon

✳ To Make

If the coconut oil is hard, set the container in a bowl of hot water for 10 minutes or so until it softens. Then place the coconut oil in a very small bowl (a custard cup works great) together with the honey and essential oil; whip together. This sweet treat is now ready to use for an evening of enjoyment!

✳ To Use

This body honey is highly spreadable; a little goes a long way. Apply anywhere you desire some sweet but slightly sticky kissing.

Caution: This formula is not latex-friendly.

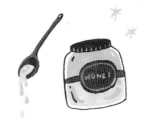

NOTE: If the temperature in your kitchen is above 76°F, the finished recipe will remain a liquid; if the temperature falls below 76°F, it will be a medium-soft solid.

Ginger–Vanilla
HONEY DRIZZLE

Is it hot in here, or is it just the ginger? Aside from being a premier digestive aid, ginger stimulates circulation and blood flow, which makes this tasty honey drizzle the perfect aphrodisiac for a night of sizzling passion!

INGREDIENTS

1 cup raw honey (liquid, not crystallized)

½ cup coarsely chopped fresh ginger

2 teaspoons vanilla extract

Makes about 1 heaping cup

BONUS: Oh yeah, it also tastes fabulous when poured over carrot cake, hot gingerbread, French toast, or pancakes, and it adds a flavor sensation when stirred into iced or hot tea, vanilla ice cream, or plain yogurt. Nothing like a multipurpose recipe!

✳ To Make

Combine the honey, ginger, and vanilla in a pint-size canning jar and stir thoroughly to blend. Cover the jar with a piece of plastic wrap and screw on the lid. Store in the refrigerator for 2 weeks, gently shaking the contents twice daily as the flavors mingle and mellow. When you add fresh ginger to thick honey, a chemical reaction occurs that dramatically thins the honey, making it more like a divinely spicy, sweet, and sticky nectar.

Strain the honey, which should be considerably thinner by now, through a fine-mesh strainer. Gently press the ginger bits with the back of a large spoon to release all the residual juice and honey. Pour the yummy syrup into a bottle, then cap, label, and store in the fridge, where it will keep for up to 3 months.

✳ To Use

Lightly drizzle this warming, luscious infusion onto any body part that you want to kiss or be kissed — lips, fingers, toes, nose, breasts, soft belly . . . let your imagination run wild!

Caution: Avoid using this honey near sensitive genital tissue, where it might sting rather than invigorate.

Soothing & Slippery Lubricants

I've never understood why commercially prepared personal lubricants contain so many harmful ingredients when there are effective natural alternatives available. Who needs those deleterious ingredients in one of the most delicate areas of the body? Every single one of the following recipes is completely edible and totally chemical-free.

They glide lovingly onto the skin, making things more fun and definitely more comfortable, especially for women suffering from vaginal dryness. They're perfect for times of sexual intimacy, encouraging closeness and awakening arousal. (Of course, while these recipes do serve as sensual, moisturizing lubricants, they should not take the place of foreplay. Natural lubrication occurs when a woman is lovingly caressed and stimulated.)

Note: These lubricants will not encourage yeast proliferation. The sweetener, if any, used in the following recipes is vegetable glycerin, which is not a desired carbohydrate food source for yeast.

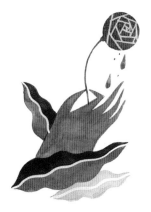

Personal Comfort
LUBRICANT CREAM

Many women experience vaginal dryness at some time or other. It can be incredibly irritating, as well as making intercourse uncomfortable, if not downright painful. I formulated this superthick cream with its pleasing scent and flavor as an ultramoisturizing personal lubricant that gently hydrates and comforts delicate tissues, both externally and internally.

INGREDIENTS

- 1 tablespoon plus 1 teaspoon sunflower or almond oil (or your favorite neutral oil)
- 1 tablespoon extra-virgin, unrefined coconut oil
- 2 teaspoons cocoa butter
- 2 teaspoons beeswax
- 1 teaspoon vegetable glycerin
- 500 IU vitamin E oil

Makes about ¼ cup

✳ To Make

Combine the sunflower oil, coconut oil, cocoa butter, beeswax, and glycerin in a small saucepan or double boiler and warm over low heat until the solids are melted. Remove from the heat and let cool for a few minutes, stirring a few times to blend. Add the vitamin E oil, then steadily beat the mixture with a spoon for a few minutes until it thickens slightly and becomes opaque. This ensures that the water-based glycerin is thoroughly incorporated.

Pour into a 2-ounce jar or tin. Cap, label, and set aside for 4 hours to let the cream synergize and thicken. Because of the coconut oil, this product will have a harder consistency at cooler temperatures and softer consistency at temperatures over 76°F. No refrigeration is required, but for maximum aroma and taste, use within 1 year.

✳ To Use

Apply as needed to lubricate and comfort dry skin and vaginal tissue. Can also be used as a lip balm, cuticle softener, and body butter.

Caution: This cream is not latex-friendly.

COCONUT OIL & COCOA BUTTER
The Ultimate Moisturizers

Organic, unrefined, extra-virgin coconut oil is used by women the world over as a safe, inexpensive, and highly effective body moisturizer and personal lubricant. It serves as a basic, simple remedy for all manner of dry skin. It soothes, softens, seals in residual moisture, and lubricates even the most delicate of tissues such as the labia, perineum, vagina, and nipples, and is completely safe to use before, during, and after giving birth.

Coconut oil is a great aid for healing dry, cracked skin anywhere on the body; it also conditions brittle nails and cuticles, relieves chapped lips, and soothes scaly patches of skin and other symptoms of dermatitis. It's a superior oil for treating and preventing blisters on your feet, and it can be used as a daily after-bath massage oil to keep your skin blissfully soft, in top condition, and smelling of rich, ripe coconuts. I even use a tiny dab to defrizz the ends of my dry, curly hair.

Cocoa butter, the oily, fragrant part of the cocoa bean, is moisturizing and comforting to dry skin. A small amount (approximately the size of a small marble) inserted into the vagina will quickly melt, adding a soothing slipperiness to dry tissues. It is generally safe to use by all women, even those with sensitivities to ordinary lubricants, and will not contribute to yeast overgrowth. In fact, no natural fatty oil or butter will encourage yeast proliferation unless a sweetener such as table sugar, fructose, honey, maple syrup, or agave nectar is added.

With both coconut oil and cocoa butter, a little goes a long way, so use them judiciously — and remember that neither is latex-friendly.

Three Cs

FEEL-GOOD OIL

Chamomile, calendula, and comfrey — the three ultra-calming, cooling, and comforting "Cs" of the herb world — contain vulnerary (tissue-healing), anti-inflammatory, mildly astringent, and emollient properties. With an amazing slip and slide on the skin, this infused oil soothes and lubricates delicate, dry intimate tissues, both internally and externally. The blend also serves as a highly penetrating and nourishing body, bath, and massage oil.

INGREDIENTS

- ½ cup dried or 1 cup fresh calendula flowers
- ½ cup dried or 1 cup fresh chamomile flowers
- ½ cup dried or 1 cup fresh comfrey leaves
- 3 cups almond, jojoba, sunflower, sesame, or extra-virgin olive oil (the latter two being the heaviest in texture and strongest in scent)
- 2,000 IU vitamin E oil

Makes about 2½ cups

✳ To Make

If you're using fresh calendula or comfrey, cut or tear the flowers or leaves into smaller pieces to expose more surface area to the oil (the chamomile flowers need no processing, as they are quite small). Combine the calendula, chamomile, and comfrey with your chosen base oil in a 2-quart saucepan or double boiler and stir thoroughly to blend. Bring the mixture to just shy of a simmer, between 125° and 135°F. Do not let the oil actually simmer — it will degrade the quality of your infused oil.

Allow the herbs to macerate (steep) in the oil over low heat, uncovered, for 5 hours. Stir the mixture and check its temperature (with a candy thermometer) every 30 minutes or so, adjusting the heat accordingly. If you're using a double boiler, add more water to the bottom as necessary, so it doesn't dry out.

After 5 hours, remove the pan from the heat and let it cool for 15 minutes. While the oil is still warm, carefully strain it through a fine-mesh strainer lined with a fine filter such as muslin or, preferably, a paper coffee filter; then strain again if necessary to remove all debris. Squeeze or press the herbs to extract as much of the precious oil as possible.

Add the vitamin E oil and stir to blend. The resulting infused oil will be a lovely hue of greenish gold-orange, varying a bit depending on which base oil you chose. Pour the oil into elegant glass storage bottles (though plastic squeeze bottles may be more convenient for use), then cap, label, and store in a dark, cool cabinet for up to 1 year.

✳ To Use

Use liberally and joyfully, any- and everywhere, to inspire natural lubrication, or apply as needed to lubricate, soothe, and comfort dry intimate tissues. Doubles as a skin-conditioning bath, body, or massage oil.

Caution: This oil is not latex-friendly.

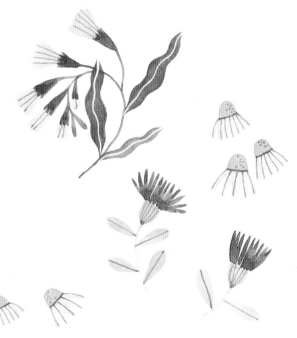

Luscious Lip Treats for Kissable Moments

Remember your first kiss? I do. I was barely 14. My heart was racing, palms sweating, stomach churning, body quivering uncontrollably in anticipation of meeting tall, lanky, wild-haired, blue-eyed, 15-year-old Mitch for our prearranged afternoon kiss down by the creek. He was going to show me how it was done by an "experienced man." Scary, yes. Exciting? You bet. When his silky-soft lips met mine, I let out a nervous scream, and he hightailed it right back up the hill from whence he came. Poor guy! I never saw him again. Makes me chuckle whenever I think about it!

The act of kissing is one of life's most wondrous, meaningful, and intimate pleasures. It can express "like," "love," or "lust" without saying a thing. And really, is there anything better than kissing for keeping romance alive?

Your lips, unlike the rest of your skin, do not contain any sebaceous (oil) or sweat glands and therefore cannot moisturize themselves; they constantly need lubrication from an outside source. Normally, a small amount of saliva combined with natural oil that seeps in from the surrounding skin is sufficient to keep them moist. However, if the lip tissue is damaged from heat, cold, matte lipsticks, dry air, smoking, sunburn, windburn, or topical or oral medications, your natural supplies of lubrication will not be sufficient to prevent your lips from becoming dry, cracked, or rough.

To keep your smoocher comfortable, conditioned, kissably soft, and inviting, try one of the following totally natural lip-pampering formulas. Take heart: all of the ingredients are edible, without a slick of petroleum jelly in sight. So pucker up, baby!

Rose-Scented Honey Lip Slick

Want lips as sweet as honey and as fragrant as a dew-kissed rose? Here's an aphrodisiacal blend that's pure ambrosia for your sultry pout! In a tiny bowl, combine 2 teaspoons of clear, raw honey with ½ teaspoon rose hydrosol or 1 drop of rose essential oil and ½ teaspoon of water. To blend, stir rapidly for about 15 seconds using a small utensil such as a chopstick or shrimp fork, or simply use your fingertip. Apply to lips immediately before sharing a tender, moist, sticky kiss with your lover.

Actually, this tasty blend can be applied anywhere you want to kiss or be kissed — it's delicious! If there's any left over, simply use it to sweeten a cup of your favorite herb tea or warm milk; it adds a most interesting flavor.

Slick 'n' Soft LIP LUBE

A basic conditioning lip balm that will enhance your kissing experience and keep your lips delectably soft and oh-so-smooth. It has a mild yet tasty almond-coconut flavor, but if left plain, it yields the subtle essence of cocoa butter and coconut — universal favorites.

INGREDIENTS

- 2 tablespoons sunflower or almond oil (or your favorite neutral oil)
- 1 tablespoon extra-virgin, unrefined coconut oil
- 2 teaspoons beeswax
- 1 teaspoon cocoa butter
- 1 drop almond flavoring oil (optional)
- 1 drop coconut flavoring oil (optional)

Makes about ¼ cup (four ½-ounce containers)

✳ To Make

Combine the base oils, beeswax, and cocoa butter in a very small saucepan or double boiler, and warm over low heat until the solids are just melted. Remove from the heat and let cool slightly for a few minutes, stirring a few times to blend. Add the flavoring oils, if desired, and stir again to thoroughly incorporate. Slowly pour the liquid lip lube into storage containers (I like ½-ounce jars or tins). Cap and label, then set aside for 4 hours to synergize and thicken completely.

For maximum aroma and taste, use within 1 year. Because of the coconut oil, this product will have a firmer consistency at cooler temperatures and softer consistency at temperatures over 76°F.

✳ To Use

To keep lips in tip-top condition, apply throughout the day, as desired, or before and after some passionate kissing.

Fruity-Minty KISSING BALM

Intensify your lip-lockin' pleasure with this silky-textured, emollient lip balm. It delivers a succulent blend of sweet fruit and mint. Note that the recipe calls for refined shea butter; you can use unrefined shea butter, but its stronger fragrance and flavor will tend to mask the fruity-minty aroma and taste.

INGREDIENTS

- 2 tablespoons plus 1 teaspoon sunflower or almond oil (or your favorite neutral oil)
- 1 teaspoon castor oil
- 2 teaspoons refined shea butter
- 1 teaspoon beeswax
- 1 teaspoon raw honey
- 8 drops sweet orange essential oil
- 4 drops spearmint essential oil

Makes about ¼ cup (four ½-ounce containers)

✳ To Make

Combine the sunflower oil, castor oil, shea butter, beeswax, and honey in a very small saucepan or double boiler and warm over low heat until the solids are just melted. Remove from the heat and let cool slightly for a few minutes, stirring a few times to blend. Add the sweet orange and spearmint essential oils, then steadily beat the mixture with a small spoon for a minute or two, until it begins to thicken slightly and becomes opaque. (This ensures that the water-based honey is thoroughly incorporated.)

Slowly pour the liquid balm into storage containers (I like ½-ounce jars or tins). Cap and label, then set aside for 4 hours to let the ingredients synergize and the balm thicken. For maximum aroma and taste, use within 1 year.

✳ To Use

To keep your lips in tip-top condition, apply throughout the day, as desired, or before and after some passionate kissing.

Variation: As a tasty alternative, use either cherry or strawberry flavoring oil instead of the sweet orange essential oil. Add the flavoring oil to taste, blending it in 1 drop at a time. A little goes a *long* way!

Cocoa-Chai "Kiss 'n' Make Up" LIP BUTTER

For a soft, comfortable, kissable smoocher, pamper your lips with this creamy, scentual, gently stimulating lip butter. Be sure to slick some on your partner's lips, too!

INGREDIENTS

- 2 tablespoons sunflower or almond oil (or your favorite neutral oil)
- 2 teaspoons castor base oil
- 1 tablespoon cocoa butter
- 1 teaspoon beeswax
- 6 drops vanilla (CO_2) essential oil
- 5 drops ginger essential oil
- 4 drops cardamom essential oil

Makes about ¼ cup
(four ½-ounce containers)

To Make

Combine the sunflower oil, castor oil, cocoa butter, and beeswax in a very small saucepan or double boiler, and warm over low heat until the solids are just melted. Remove from the heat and let cool slightly for a few minutes, stirring a few times to blend. Add the vanilla, ginger, and cardamom essential oils and stir again to thoroughly incorporate.

Slowly pour the liquid lip butter into storage containers (I like ½-ounce jars or tins). Cap and label, then set aside for 6 hours to synergize and thicken completely. For maximum aroma and taste, use within 1 year.

To Use

To keep lips in tip-top condition, apply throughout the day, as desired, or before and after some passionate kissing.

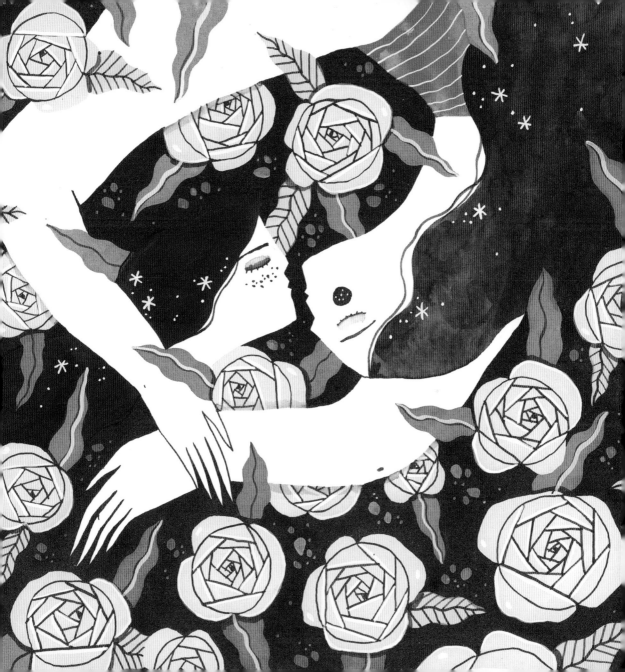

Tongue-Tantalizing
BREATH FRESHENERS

Nothing can ruin a potentially intimate moment quicker than bad breath. It's not only unpleasant for your partner but embarrassing for you, too. A lose-lose situation. If you ever find yourself in need of fresh breath in a pinch and want to skip the synthetically flavored breath mints and gum, try these natural and flavorful tips:

* **ESSENTIAL OIL BREATH DROPS.** I generally keep a tiny 5 ml bottle of peppermint essential oil in my purse for times when I need to freshen my breath quickly. Just one drop on my tongue, and I'm done! Minty-fresh breath in a snap! If peppermint isn't to your liking, try using other flavorful, odor-eliminating essential oils, such as spearmint, sweet orange, or fennel. Simply place one (and only one) drop directly on your tongue. If the flavor is too strong, immediately swish your mouth with water and spit it out.

* **FLAVORFUL SPICES.** Chew on a few fennel, anise, or cardamom seeds or suck on a whole clove or piece of candied ginger. These pungent spices will neutralize bad breath, and they help relieve gas and upset stomach — two notorious producers of offensive breath. Of these spices, cardamom seeds are my favorite, and I usually keep a tiny container of them stashed in my purse.

* **COMMERCIAL CHLOROPHYLL DROPS.** Chlorophyll is the green pigment found in plants; it acts as a natural breath sweetener and digestive aid.

* **GARNISHES.** After a garlicky or onion-laden meal, eat a sprig of parsley, watercress, or rosemary. There's a reason they're often served as a garnish! They're not just for decoration; they really help eliminate unpleasant lingering food odors and improve digestion. A lemon wedge or peppermint leaf will do the same.

* **APPLES.** Whenever you feel the need for a bit of breath cleansing, take a few bites of a crisp apple and chew very, very well. This naturally fibrous, juicy, sweet fruit whisks away odor and leaves your mouth feeling wonderfully fresh.

* **HERBAL TEAS.** Skip the coffee and black tea. These two beverages tend to astringe the mouth and leave a lingering bad taste and fuzzy, dry mouthfeel. Opt instead for a cup of strong, refreshing peppermint, ginger, fennel, or spiced chai tea. In addition to freshening your mouth and cleansing your palate, these herbal beverages serve as digestive aids, helping to prevent gas and bloating.

* **RINSE.** Swish bottled water in your mouth for at least 10 seconds, then swallow. Repeat. Then drink at least another cup. This helps loosen any food debris and moistens your mouth and throat. A moist mouth harbors less odor-causing bacteria than a dry, pasty one.

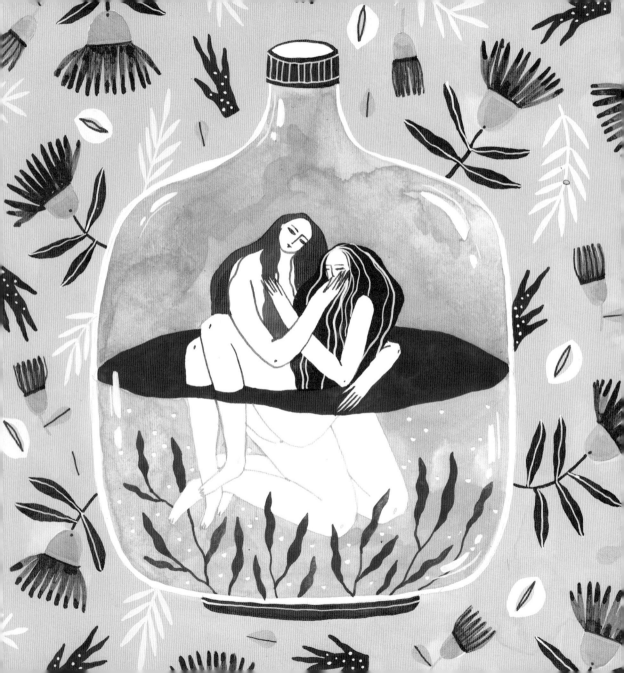

CHAPTER 6

Love Potions

Herbal Tonics to Inspire Passion

"WOO-HOO," I HEAR YOU SAYING. "Love potions — just what my sex life needs!" Now, now, calm down — don't get all hot and bothered by the title of this chapter. I'm not going to give you recipes for "magical potions" or "herbal love drugs" that will quickly transform your blasé spouse or partner into a searing, passionate love god or goddess. We mere mortals do not possess that kind of magic!

These tasty formulations are instead designed to act as restorative, adaptogenic tonics that, when taken consistently, will build warmth in your core, lubricate and moisten dry tissues, help balance hormones, strengthen immunity, nourish you deep down, enhance well-being and overall vitality, relax tensions, and relieve fatigue, thus supporting a healthy sexual appetite and giving you the necessary robust energy so you are able to make love when you want to make love.

Just what is an adaptogen, you ask? You'll see this word mentioned several times throughout this chapter.

Adaptogens help the human body adapt to stress, restore balance, and support normal metabolic processes. They increase the body's resistance to biological, physical, emotional, and environmental stressors and promote normal physiologic function. In the past they have been called rejuvenating herbs, rasayanas, restoratives, and chi (energy) tonics, and they have a long tradition of being superior healing herbs. The wide range of health benefits they offer covers almost every area of the body, which is why I use them in these nourishing recipes.

If your "get up and go" got up and went, the recipes in this chapter are just what you need to replenish and balance your being.

If you've been doing too much, giving too much, neglecting yourself, and feeling exhausted, stressed out, and frazzled, and your love life has taken a backseat because your "get up and go" got up and went, the recipes in this chapter are just what you need to replenish and balance your being. Keep in mind that these formulations are herbal supplements and work best when combined with a healthy diet and lifestyle.

Rejuvenative
BANANA-YOGURT SMOOTHIE

Feeling stressed out, frazzled, and fatigued? This smoothie has shatavari and astragalus roots, two rejuvenating herbs that combine to help the body adapt to stress. They also soothe an irritated digestive tract and sore, achy joints and muscles. This creamy, mildly sweet-tart concoction will help enhance overall well-being and vitality, strengthen the immune system, and gently energize without overstimulating. It makes a tasty, filling breakfast, lunch, or late afternoon pick-me-up.

INGREDIENTS

- 2 cups plain yogurt (whole milk or low fat, your choice), preferably organic
- 1 cup water
- 2 medium fresh or frozen bananas, cut into chunks
- 2 tablespoons raw honey, raw agave nectar, or maple syrup
- 2 teaspoons vanilla extract
- ½ teaspoon ground cinnamon
- ½ teaspoon shatavari root powder
- ½ teaspoon astragalus root powder

Makes 2 servings

✳ To Make

Combine the yogurt, water, bananas, honey, vanilla, cinnamon, shatavari, and astragalus in a blender and blend on high until smooth, about 30 seconds.

✳ To Use

Pour into chilled tumblers or insulated mugs. This blend has moderate levels of natural sugars, fats, and fiber; sip slowly so you can digest it with ease. Let the rejuvenation begin . . .

Spicy Cocoa-Maca
SMOOTHIE

Both cocoa beans and maca root, high in minerals and other valuable phytonutrients, have been revered for thousands of years by South American Indians as longevity foods that promote strength and endurance, boost immunity, and improve libido. This smoothie tastes like a chocolate-banana malted with the added bite of warming, circulation-enhancing cayenne pepper and cinnamon. This delicious combo is a great treat to share with your honey!

INGREDIENTS

1½ cups water

2 medium or 3 small bananas, cut into chunks

4 tablespoons almond or cashew butter, raw or roasted

1 tablespoon raw cocoa (cacao) powder or natural unsweetened cocoa

1 tablespoon raw honey, raw agave nectar, or maple syrup

2 teaspoons maca root powder

1 teaspoon vanilla extract

¼ teaspoon ground cayenne

¼ teaspoon ground cinnamon

Pinch of sea salt

Makes 2 servings

✳ To Make

Combine the water, bananas, nut butter, cocoa, honey, maca, vanilla, cayenne, cinnamon, and salt in a blender and blend on high until smooth, about 30 seconds.

✳ To Use

Serve in chilled tumblers or insulated mugs. This blend is high in natural sugars, fats, and fiber; sip slowly so you can digest it with ease. Feel the spicy energy coursing through your veins!

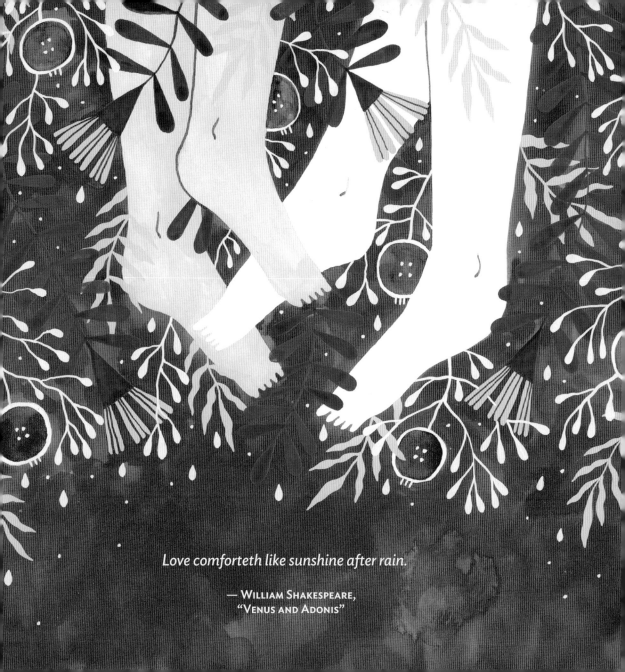

Love comforteth like sunshine after rain.

— WILLIAM SHAKESPEARE,
"VENUS AND ADONIS"

DAMIANA-GINGER-SCHISANDRA *Elixir*

A sweet, potent, smooth blend of warming, flavorful, restorative herbs that will increase circulation throughout the body, enhance functioning of the immune system, treat frigidity in women and impotence in men, balance the nervous system, improve digestion, and serve as a gentle chi or energy tonic (among other benefits). A wonderful tonic for those who feel physically and mentally exhausted.

INGREDIENTS

- 1 cup good-quality 80-proof brandy
- ½ cup raw honey
- 2 teaspoons vanilla extract
- ½ cup finely chopped fresh ginger
- 1 tablespoon damiana leaf powder (or 3 tablespoons dried, crushed leaves)
- 1 tablespoon schisandra berry powder (or 3 tablespoons dried berries)
- 2 cinnamon sticks

Makes about 1¼ cups

✳ To Make

Combine the brandy, honey, and vanilla in a pint-size canning jar, then add the ginger, damiana, schisandra, and cinnamon sticks. Cover the jar with a piece of plastic wrap and screw on the lid. Shake the mixture vigorously for 15 seconds to blend. Store the jar in a cool, dark place for 4 weeks, shaking the contents daily as the flavors mingle and mellow.

Strain the elixir through a fine-mesh strainer lined with a fine filter such as muslin or, preferably, a paper coffee filter; then strain again if necessary to remove all herb debris. Press or squeeze the herbs to release all the valuable herbal extract. Pour the lovely reddish-amber elixir into an elegant glass storage bottle, then cap, label, and store in a dark, cool cabinet for up to 6 months.

✷ To Use

Enjoy as a sipping beverage as desired. To use it as a restorative tonic, take 1 teaspoon of elixir per day for 3 to 4 weeks, discontinue for 1 week, then repeat the cycle. Simply add it to your favorite hot tea (chai is great) or warm milk, or just take it straight, followed by a few sips of water.

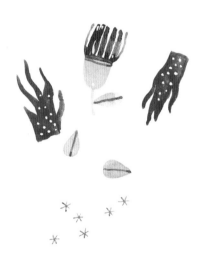

Enjoying Your Elixirs

Aphrodite's Lucky-in-Love Liqueur (page 102) and Damiana-Ginger-Schisandra Elixir (page 100) are both potent and delicious love potions. For a wonderfully relaxing and arousing evening, pour your chilled homemade elixir into two beautiful, slender stemware glasses and share with your lover. But enjoy these delightful drinks in moderation, lest you become too relaxed to enjoy the passionate evening ahead!

You might also try delicately drizzling these nectars onto your lover's body for some tasty fun. Or drizzle them over sliced ripe strawberries, peaches, and bananas and cubes of rich pound cake for a sinfully delicious dessert.

Aphrodite's Lucky-in-Love
LIQUEUR

This love liqueur is gently powerful, warm, and spicy-sweet. Eleuthero is revered for increasing sexual and physical endurance, stamina, energy, and resistance to all types of stress. Spicy, biting ginger has been shown to stimulate circulation and impart warmth to your core, then radiate that heat to the extremities.

INGREDIENTS

½ cup good-quality 80-proof brandy

½ cup good-quality 80-proof vodka

½ cup water

¼ cup raw honey

2 tablespoons chopped dried eleuthero root

1 tablespoon diced dried or candied ginger (or 2 tablespoons fresh)

½ teaspoon cardamom seeds

10–15 dried, pitted tart cherries (optional, but delicious)

6 small dried or candied apricots, diced

1 cinnamon stick

1 vanilla bean, sliced lengthwise and cut into ½-inch pieces

Makes about 1½ cups

✳ To Make

Combine the brandy, vodka, water, honey, eleuthero, ginger, cardamom, cherries (if using), apricots, cinnamon stick, and vanilla bean in a pint-size (or larger) canning jar with a tight-fitting lid. Cover the jar with a piece of plastic wrap and screw on the lid. Shake the mixture vigorously for 15 seconds to blend. Store the jar in a cool, dark place for 4 weeks, shaking the contents daily as the flavors mingle and mellow.

Strain the liquid through a fine-mesh strainer. Bottle and store in the refrigerator, where the liqueur will keep for 3 months.

✳ To Use

Enjoy as a sipping beverage as desired. Or, as a restorative tonic, take 1 teaspoon of liqueur per day for 3 to 4 weeks, discontinue for 1 week, then repeat the cycle. Simply add to your favorite hot tea or warm milk, or just take it straight followed by a few sips of water.

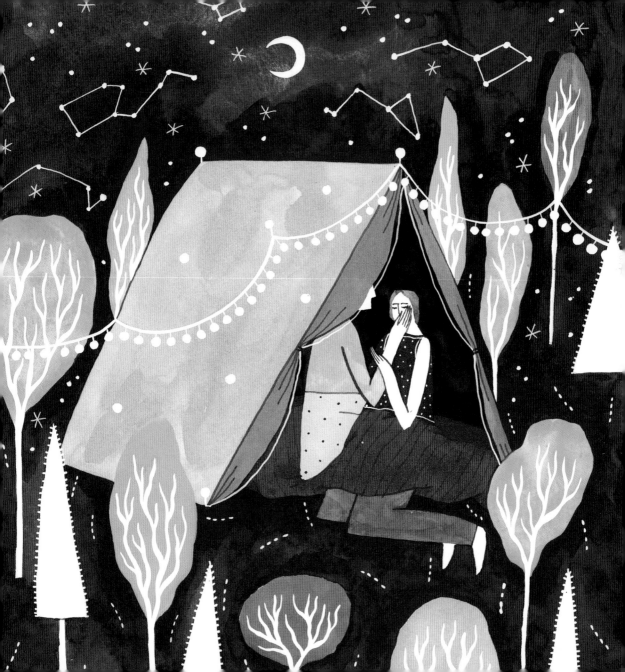

Schi-Zaam SCHISANDRA & GINSENG HARMONIZING HERBAL WINE

This delectable red-wine infusion of five-flavored schisandra berries and American ginseng root is an adaptogenic, restorative tonic brew that, with regular consumption, will help harmonize your physiological systems to increase your resistance to the damaging effects of disease and stress, build core energy and stamina, boost sex drive, enhance cognitive function, improve cardiovascular health, and promote longevity.

INGREDIENTS

- ½ cup dried schisandra berries
- 2 medium dried American ginseng roots (each about the size of a woman's pinkie), or 3 tablespoons chopped dried eleuthero root
- 1 bottle fine red wine, preferably organic

Makes about 3 cups

✳ To Make

Combine the schisandra berries and ginseng roots in a 1-quart canning jar. Pour the wine over them, to within ½ inch of the top. Wash and save the wine bottle; you'll need it as the final storage container. Cover the jar with a piece of plastic wrap and screw on the lid. Shake the mixture vigorously for 15 seconds to blend. Let the brew steep in a cool, dark place for 4 weeks; over this time the wine will extract valuable chemical components from the herbs and the flavors will develop. Shake the jar for 15 to 30 seconds each day.

Remove the ginseng roots, cut them into thin slivers, and set aside. Strain the wine through a fine-mesh strainer lined with a fine filter, such as muslin or, preferably, a paper coffee filter; then strain again if necessary to remove all the herb debris. Press or squeeze the berries to wring out all the valuable herbal extract. Pour the wine back into the original bottle and toss in the ginseng root slivers. Then cap, label, and store in the refrigerator for up to 3 months.

✳ To Use

Enjoy a glass of infused wine with your partner in the evening; it's a great way to unwind after a stressful day. Or to use it as a restorative herbal tonic, drink ⅓ cup daily for 3 to 4 weeks, discontinue for 1 week, then repeat the cycle. This brew tantalizes the taste buds, delivering the complete spectrum of flavors: sweet, sour, salty, pungent, and bitter. Sip it very slowly, and enjoy the sensory explosion!

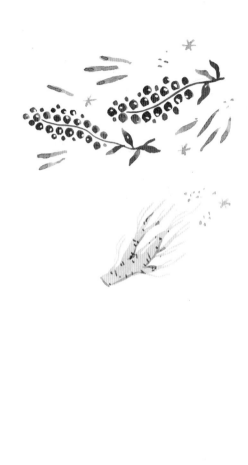

Electuaries: Herbal Honey Pastes

Never heard of an electuary? Well, then you've been missing out on a most pleasant way of ingesting healing herbs. Electuaries have been used for thousands of years as a sweet and tasty delivery vehicle for medicinal herbs. They're made simply by blending either powdered or very finely ground herbs and spices with honey; the result is a sweet paste that can be eaten right off the spoon. Hippocrates said, "Your food should be your medicine, and your medicine your food," and electuaries are sweet medicinal food indeed!

Electuaries act as herbal supplements. If you eat them consistently, twice daily to start, you should begin to feel the benefits within a few weeks, if not sooner, provided you observe healthy diet and lifestyle habits. The following three recipes are my favorites. Give one a try, won't you?

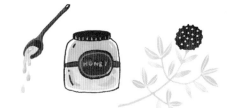

"Vital Man" ELECTUARY

Vital Man is a restorative, tonic, adaptogenic blend formulated for men over 40. It increases endurance, strength, vitality, and deep core energy without being overly stimulating. It is chock-full of the yang life force needed for male reproductive, prostate, adrenal, kidney, and liver health and, when taken consistently over a period of time, should improve virility and sexual energy.

INGREDIENTS

- 2 tablespoons eleuthero root powder (or American ginseng, if unavailable)
- 1 tablespoon ashwagandha root powder
- 1 tablespoon astragalus root powder
- 1 tablespoon ground cinnamon
- 1 tablespoon fo-ti root powder
- 1 tablespoon maca root powder
- 1 tablespoon saw palmetto berry powder
- 1 cup raw honey (liquid, not crystallized)

Makes about 1 cup

CONTRAINDICATION

Any woman considering this energizing formula should not consume it if she is pregnant or nursing.

✴ To Make

Combine the eleuthero, ashwagandha, astragalus, cinnamon, fo-ti, maca, and saw palmetto in a bowl and mix well. Stir in ½ cup of the honey. Gradually stir in more honey until a very soft, thick paste forms. Store in a tightly sealed container in the refrigerator for 24 hours prior to consuming to allow the medicinal properties to synergize and the flavors to develop; keep refrigerated and use within 3 months.

✴ To Use

As a supplement, take ½ teaspoon twice daily for 3 weeks, then take 1 week off. Repeat the sequence as desired until you begin to feel better, then cut back to ½ teaspoon per day. You may eat the electuary directly from the spoon, stir it into hot herb tea or warm milk, or spread it on a sturdy cracker. The flavor should be sweet, spicy, warm, rooty, and pungent, with the predominant taste coming from the ever-so-beneficial, yet rather distasteful, saw palmetto berries, which I've tried to camouflage among the other herbs.

"Keep Life Juicy" WOMEN'S RESTORATIVE ELECTUARY

This warming, tonic, adaptogenic blend — especially recommended for women over 40 who are feeling frazzled and deficient — slowly increases overall vitality, endurance, and stamina. Taken consistently over time, this formula will assist in lubricating and soothing the body's tissues, toning the female reproductive system, balancing hormones, supporting liver and adrenal health, and enhancing sexual energy. Being a primarily root-based formulation, it will have a grounding effect on the psyche and nervous system, thereby restoring a sense of calm and promoting sound sleep.

INGREDIENTS

- 2 tablespoons shatavari root powder
- 1 tablespoon ashwagandha root powder
- 1 tablespoon astragalus root powder
- 1 tablespoon eleuthero root powder (or American ginseng, if unavailable)
- 1 tablespoon fo-ti root powder
- 1 tablespoon ground ginger
- 1 tablespoon schisandra berry powder
- About 1 cup raw honey (liquid, not crystallized)

Makes about 1 cup

✳ To Make

Combine the shatavari, ashwagandha, astragalus, eleuthero, fo-ti, ginger, and schisandra in a bowl and mix well. Stir in ½ cup of the honey. Gradually stir in more honey until a very soft, thick paste forms. Store in a tightly sealed container in the refrigerator for 24 hours prior to consuming to allow the medicinal properties to synergize and the flavors to develop; keep refrigerated and use within 3 months.

✳ To Use

As a supplement, take ½ teaspoon twice daily for 3 weeks, then take 1 week off. Repeat the sequence as desired until you begin to feel better, then cut back to ½ teaspoon per day. You may eat the electuary directly from the spoon (like I do), stir it into hot herb tea or warm milk, or spread it on a sturdy cracker. The flavor should be sweet, rooty, spicy, and slightly sour/tart, with the predominant taste coming from the schisandra berries.

CONTRAINDICATION
Do not consume if you are pregnant or nursing.

Electuary Taffy?

When you combine powdered herbs with honey, the herbs absorb a great deal of moisture from the honey. If you don't add enough honey to your electuary mixture, within 12 to 24 hours it may develop an almost taffylike consistency from the swelling of the herbs. That's okay, but just be cognizant of that fact and add more honey next time you make a fresh batch.

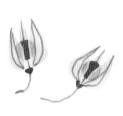

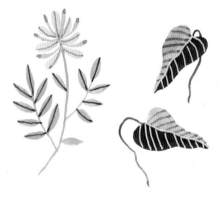

Stephanie's Love Potion #8:
CACAO-KAVA ELECTUARY

This tasty electuary looks like thick, shiny chocolate syrup and provides a bevy of benefits for both men and women. If taken consistently over time, it increases lubrication throughout the body, helping to reduce inflammation and dryness. It also promotes endurance, strength, vitality, and deep core energy, without being overly stimulating; helps maintain beauty and youthfulness; delivers a balancing energy to the reproductive system; and has a grounding effect on the psyche and nervous system, leaving you calm but still quite alert.

INGREDIENTS

- 2 tablespoons raw cocoa (cacao) powder or natural unsweetened cocoa powder
- 2 tablespoons maca root powder
- 1 tablespoon eleuthero root powder (or American ginseng, if unavailable)
- 1 tablespoon shatavari root powder
- 2 teaspoons ground cinnamon

- 2 teaspoons damiana leaf powder
- 2 teaspoons kava-kava root powder
- 2 tablespoons vanilla extract
- ¾–1 cup raw honey (liquid, not crystallized; use the greater amount for a softer consistency)

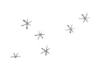

Makes about 1 cup

✳ To Make

Combine the cocoa, maca, eleuthero, shatavari, cinnamon, damiana, and kava-kava in a medium bowl and mix with a small whisk or spoon. Add the vanilla, followed by the honey, and stir thoroughly to blend. It should look like thick, shiny chocolate syrup. Store in a tightly sealed, labeled, dated container in the refrigerator for 24 hours prior to consuming to allow the medicinal properties to synergize and flavors to develop; keep refrigerated and use within 3 months.

CONTRAINDICATION

This formulation is not to be consumed by women who are pregnant or nursing, or anyone with liver problems. Because of the kava-kava, consuming this electuary in excess — over the recommended amounts — may impair your ability to drive or operate heavy machinery. It is also not recommended for consumption with alcoholic beverages.

✳ To Use

As a supplement, take ½ teaspoon twice daily for 3 weeks, then take 1 week off. Repeat the sequence as desired until you begin to feel better, then cut back to ½ teaspoon per day. You may eat the electuary directly from the spoon, stir it into hot herb tea or warm milk, or spread it on a cracker, cookie, or piece of raw, sharp cheese (yum!). The flavor should be sweet, spicy, rich, and chocolaty, with hints of malt and a pungent note that jumps out from the damiana and kava-kava. It's quite scrumptious — an herbal supplement you'll look forward to taking!

This is a wonderful formula to take for the enhancement of sexual energy and heightened mental awareness. A formulation that stirs the cauldron of passion within and ignites love's flame, it's a definite herbal aphrodisiac if there ever was one — it even makes the tongue tingle!

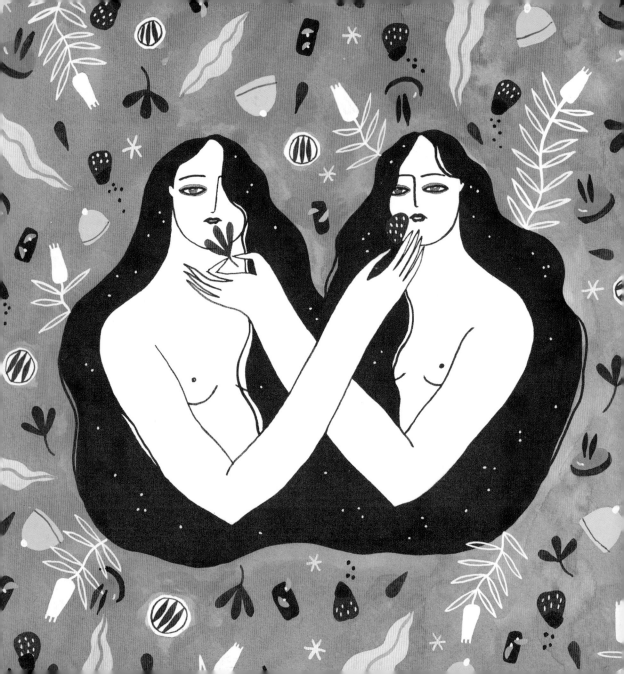

CHAPTER 7

Delectably Decadent
SWEETS

AS FAR AS I'M CONCERNED, I've saved the best recipes for last. These edible "sweet seductions" are designed to be nibbled slowly, shared, and savored. A sweet finger-food feast can be a highly erotic adventure — you never know where it may lead! I'm a raw food enthusiast, and most of the ingredients used here are just that: raw, unprocessed, and overflowing with grounding and building whole-food nutrition. No guilt here, just pure gustatory pleasure. Every recipe is easy to make, requires no baking, and is free of gluten, refined sugar, soy, peanuts, corn, and eggs. Most are dairy-free, too. So enjoy these extraordinarily scrumptious taste sensations — and be sure to share them with your beloved!

Macho Man

BRAZIL-NUT BALLS

These filling, rather creamy, sweet-tart energy balls are high in zinc and selenium, essential nutrients for the sexually active man, and I've added maca root for its libido- and stamina-enhancing properties. Women love them, too, as regular consumption will boost energy, encourage luxurious growth of hair and nails, and promote clear skin.

INGREDIENTS

- 1 cup finely shredded unsweetened coconut
- ½ cup raw cocoa (cacao) powder or natural unsweetened cocoa powder
- 2 cups raw Brazil nuts
- 1 cup dried cranberries, sweetened or unsweetened
- ¼ cup raw pumpkin seeds (pepitas)
- 1 tablespoon maca root powder
- 2 teaspoons ground cinnamon
  Pinch of sea salt
- ½ cup raw honey or agave nectar

Makes about 25 balls

✳ To Make

Set aside ½ cup of the shredded coconut and the cocoa powder in separate shallow bowls for coating the balls. Combine the remaining ½ cup coconut with the Brazil nuts, cranberries, pumpkin seeds, maca powder, cinnamon, and salt in a food processor and blend until you have a nutty, granular consistency, about 30 seconds. Add the honey and blend again until you achieve a slightly sticky, moist, oily, semicohesive dough, about 60 seconds.

Scrape the dough into a large bowl. For each ball, scoop out a walnut-size portion of the dough. The dough will be soft and a bit crumbly; squeeze it in your hand into a ball about 1¼ inches in diameter. Set the balls on waxed paper. Roll half of them in the cocoa powder and half in the shredded coconut to coat.

For the best flavor and firmer consistency, let the balls chill in the refrigerator for 24 hours before eating. Store in a tightly sealed container in the refrigerator and consume within 2 to 3 weeks. Alternatively, you can store them in the freezer for up to 3 months.

HERBAL
Energy Balls

These toothsome snacks are full of vigor-building nutrients and antioxidants. The gently stimulating herbs and spices combine with sweet, creamy, tart flavors to provide sustained energy in one small package. Herbalists recommend taking eleuthero on a regular basis to increase stamina and endurance and restore vitality deep within your core.

INGREDIENTS

- 1 cup finely shredded unsweetened coconut
- 1 cup almond butter or sesame tahini, raw or roasted
- ¾ cup dried cranberries, sweetened or unsweetened
- ½ cup raw honey
- 2 tablespoons eleuthero root powder
- ½ teaspoon ground cinnamon
  Pinch of sea salt

Makes about 20 balls

✳ To Make

Set aside ½ cup of the coconut in a shallow bowl for coating. Combine the remaining ½ cup coconut with the almond butter, cranberries, honey, eleuthero, cinnamon, and salt in a medium bowl and stir well to blend. I normally use my hands instead of a spoon to really knead the ingredients into a cohesive ball.

Pinch off pieces of the dough and form them into balls about 1¼ inches in diameter. Rinse and dry your hands periodically if they get too sticky. Roll each ball in the reserved coconut to coat and set aside on waxed paper.

For the best flavor and firmer consistency, let the balls chill in the refrigerator for 24 hours before eating. Store in a tightly sealed container in the refrigerator and consume within 2 to 3 weeks, or store in the freezer for up to 3 months. They may be individually wrapped, using waxed paper or plastic wrap, and taken with you to enjoy as portable energy bites.

Sweet Ginger
BUZZ BALLS

If you adore the hot, stimulating bite of ginger, then you'll love these soft, gooey, rich confections infused with stamina- and vitality-building, rejuvenating, stress-reducing, libido-enhancing, longevity-boosting, deeply nourishing herbs and bee pollen. They make great "kissing treats," as they leave a lingering, spicy-sweet taste in your mouth.

INGREDIENTS

- 1¼ cups raw almonds
- ½ cup crystallized ginger pieces
- ⅓ cup raw honey
- 4 tablespoons bee pollen
- 1 tablespoon eleuthero root powder
- 1 tablespoon fo-ti root powder
- ¼ teaspoon sea salt
- Raw, unrefined coconut oil
- ½ cup finely shredded unsweetened coconut

Makes about 28 balls

✳ To Make

Grind the almonds to the consistency of a medium- to fine-grained meal in a food processor or nut and seed grinder. Dice the crystallized ginger into ¼-inch cubes. Transfer the almond meal and diced ginger to a medium bowl and add the honey, bee pollen, eleuthero, fo-ti, and sea salt. Use your hands to mash all the ingredients together until a semicohesive ball forms. The dough should be very sticky. If it's too dry, add a little more honey; if it's too moist, grind and add a little more almond meal.

Oil your hands well with coconut oil. Pinch off pieces of dough, roll them into marble-size balls about 1 inch in diameter, and set them aside on waxed paper. Re-oil your hands as necessary. Put the shredded coconut in a shallow bowl and roll each ball in the coconut to coat.

For the best flavor and consistency, let the balls chill in the refrigerator for 24 hours before eating. Store in a tightly sealed container in the refrigerator and consume within 2 or 3 weeks, or store in the freezer for up to 3 months.

MEXICAN DARK CHOCOLATE-BLUEBERRY *Divine Fudge*

Experience raw candy decadence at its finest! If you're familiar with the taste of Mexican chocolate, then you know it can have a pungent bite. This unique fudge has plenty of tongue-tantalizing flavors and textures: bitter and sweet, hot and rich, smooth and chewy, melt-in-your-mouth gooey! With regular consumption of this luscious, nutrient-packed confection, you'll see an increase in outer glow and feel a surge of inner vitality. It's a must-have sweet treat for date night!

INGREDIENTS

- ½ cup raw, unrefined coconut oil
- 1 cup dried blueberries, sweetened with apple juice or unsweetened
- 1 cup raw cocoa (cacao) powder or natural unsweetened cocoa powder
- ½ cup almond butter, raw or roasted
- 2 tablespoons raw honey or agave nectar
- 1 teaspoon chili powder
- 1 teaspoon ground cinnamon
- ½ teaspoon ground cayenne
- ¼ teaspoon sea salt

Makes about 24 pieces

✳ To Make

If the coconut oil is solid, set the jar in a pan of very hot water or in a warm, sunny window to liquefy. Combine the coconut oil, blueberries, cocoa, almond butter, honey, chili powder, cinnamon, cayenne, and salt in a large bowl and stir to blend until a stiff ball forms. There will be small lumps of blueberries.

Coat the bottom of an 8-inch square pan with coconut oil or line with waxed paper. Spread the fudge mixture in the pan to an approximate depth of 1 inch. Cover and freeze for 1 hour, until very firm. Then remove from the freezer and let the mixture soften slightly for about 20 minutes. Cut the fudge into 1½-inch squares.

Store in a tightly sealed container in the refrigerator for up to 2 months or in the freezer for up to 6 months. Do not allow the fudge to sit at room temperature for too long or it will melt.

Dark Chocolate-Cinnamon
TURTLES

This raw, melt-in-your-mouth version of the classic "chocolate turtle" confection is sure to please. Oh-so-rich and fudgy with a bite of warming cinnamon — the perfect bittersweet treat to share with your lover after dinner or an evening of passion. It's wonderful accompanied by a hot cup of chai tea or cold vanilla rice or almond milk. Yum!

INGREDIENTS

- ½ cup almond butter, raw or roasted
- ½ cup raw cocoa (cacao) powder or natural unsweetened cocoa powder
- ¼ cup raw honey or agave nectar
- 2 teaspoons ground cinnamon
- Pinch of sea salt
- 16 raw pecan halves

Makes about 16 pieces

✳ To Make

Combine the almond butter, cocoa, honey, cinnamon, and salt in a medium bowl and slowly stir to blend until a slightly sticky, dark, stiff dough forms. Line the bottom of an 8-inch square pan with parchment or waxed paper. Pinch off pieces of the dough and roll into balls about 1 inch in diameter. Rinse and dry your hands periodically if they get too sticky. Set the balls in the pan so they are not touching.

Gently press a pecan half into the top of each ball, flattening slightly. Cover the pan and chill in the refrigerator for at least 4 hours prior to consuming. They'll become a little firmer but will still be pleasantly soft. I prefer to store and eat them directly out of the freezer, as they become quite firm but still chewy, and the pecan gets crunchy. Whichever method you choose, always store your turtles in a tightly sealed container; they'll keep in the refrigerator for up to 3 weeks and in the freezer for up to 3 months.

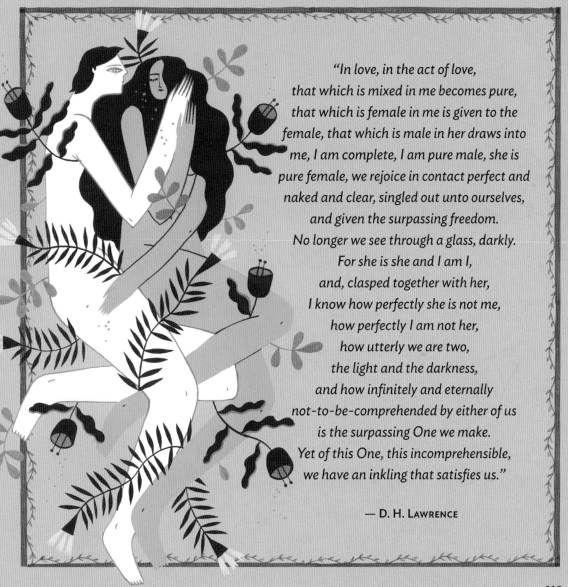

"In love, in the act of love,
that which is mixed in me becomes pure,
that which is female in me is given to the
female, that which is male in her draws into
me, I am complete, I am pure male, she is
pure female, we rejoice in contact perfect and
naked and clear, singled out unto ourselves,
and given the surpassing freedom.
No longer we see through a glass, darkly.
For she is she and I am I,
and, clasped together with her,
I know how perfectly she is not me,
how perfectly I am not her,
how utterly we are two,
the light and the darkness,
and how infinitely and eternally
not-to-be-comprehended by either of us
is the surpassing One we make.
Yet of this One, this incomprehensible,
we have an inkling that satisfies us."

— D. H. LAWRENCE

Vegan
DARK CHOCOLATE SYRUP

This decadently dark, sinfully rich yet healthful syrup can be enjoyed in many ways: drizzled over fresh pear or banana slices or pieces of moist lemon pound cake; used as a dip for juicy, ripe strawberries; stirred into warm milk; or lightly spread any place on your partner's body that you want to sweetly kiss. It's amazingly lip-smackin' good!

INGREDIENTS

- 1 teaspoon raw, unre-fined coconut oil
- 3 tablespoons raw honey or agave nectar
- 2 tablespoons raw cocoa (cacao) powder or natural unsweetened cocoa powder
- ¼ teaspoon vanilla extract
  Dash of ground cinnamon
  Pinch of sea salt

Makes about ⅓ cup

✳ To Make

If the coconut oil is solid, set the container in a pan of very hot water or in a warm, sunny window to liquefy. Combine the coconut oil, honey, cocoa, vanilla, cinnamon, and salt in a small bowl and stir vigorously to blend. The mixture should resemble a rather thick chocolate syrup.

Store the syrup in a tightly sealed container and refrigerate for up to 3 weeks, but it probably won't last that long!

NOTE: The syrup will become almost firm if chilled. To soften, simply set the bowl in a shallow pan of warm water for 10 minutes.

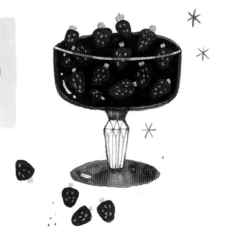

DARK CHOCOLATE–COCONUT
Bliss Fondue

Entice your beloved with a luscious, thick, chocolaty taste sensation that's out of this world! This deep, seductive sauce provides a titillating, sweet indulgence that should be enjoyed slowly and savored . . . just like a romantic evening.

INGREDIENTS

- ½ cup raw, unrefined coconut oil
- 1 cup raw cocoa (cacao) powder or natural unsweetened cocoa powder
- ¾ cup raw honey or agave nectar
- ½ teaspoon ground cinnamon
- ¼ teaspoon sea salt
  Finger foods for dipping, as desired

Makes about 1¾ cups

✳ To Make

If the coconut oil is solid, set the container in a pan of very hot water or in a sunny window to liquefy. Combine the coconut oil, cocoa, honey, cinnamon, and salt in a medium bowl and whisk together until very smooth and quite thick.

Scrape out the gooey fondue into a small, pretty bowl. Place the bowl of fondue in the center of a beautiful dessert platter and surround it with an array of yummy finger foods that pair well with chocolate (see the suggestions at right). Dip as desired. Have fun with it!

Store any leftovers in a small, tightly sealed container in the refrigerator for up to 3 weeks. When chilled, it will become very dense and fudgelike. To soften, leave covered at warm room temperature for 2 or 3 hours.

Variation: To make a healthy version of Nutella, try blending ½ cup of fondue with ½ cup of raw or roasted almond butter — utterly delish!

FONDUE FINGER FOODS

Banana and pear slices

Biscotti

Dried or candied apricots

Fresh pineapple chunks

Crystallized or candied ginger or orange peel

Sharp cheddar cheese cubes

Sweet strawberries

Walnuts and Brazil nuts

Sweet Yogurt CHEESE

If you've never tried sweet yogurt cheese before, then you're in for a delicious surprise. It's creamy, thick, and smooth — a bit softer than cream cheese — and easily infused with the flavors of spices, natural sweeteners, dried fruit, fruit juice, and citrus zest. If you're fond of soft cheeses, try these two easy-to-make recipes.

Sweet Vanilla–Orange

INGREDIENTS

- 1 quart organic, vanilla-flavored, whole-milk yogurt (do not use Greek-style)
- ¼ cup orange juice concentrate, thawed
  Zest from 1 medium orange, tangerine, or tangelo (about 2 teaspoons grated)

Sweet Honey–Cinnamon

INGREDIENTS

- 1 quart organic, plain, whole-milk yogurt (do not use Greek-style)
- ¼ cup raw honey
- 1 teaspoon vanilla extract
- 1 teaspoon ground cinnamon

Makes about 2 cups

✳ To Make

Line a plastic or metal colander with several layers of cheesecloth or a linen kitchen towel. Set the colander into a slightly smaller bowl so there is a minimum of 1½ inches of space between the bottom of the colander and bottom of the bowl (this is where the liquid whey will collect as it drains from the yogurt).

Scoop the yogurt into the lined colander, then gently fold over the edges of the cloth so it covers the yogurt. Place the bowl in the refrigerator and allow the whey to drip out for at least 8 to 12 hours. The longer it drains, the thicker and richer the cheese.

When the yogurt is ready, lift the colander from the bowl and set it in the sink. Pour the slightly tart, acidophilus-rich whey into a glass, and drink it straight or and add it to a smoothie later in the day.

Open the cloth and scoop the thick mound of cheese into a medium bowl. Stir in the flavoring ingredients until thoroughly blended. Cover and refrigerate for several hours before serving so the flavors can mingle. For best taste and consistency, use within 3 days.

Variation: For a richer, sweeter flavor and wonderful chewy texture, stir in ½ cup currants or chopped, pitted dates. It's really yummy!

A Versatile Treat

Yogurt cheese can be enjoyed by the spoonful (which is my favorite way to eat it) or spread on anything from scones and fudgy brownies to apple or pear slices, sprouted bagels, multigrain toast, and crackers. Try stirring some into your breakfast oatmeal. A dollop spooned into parfait glasses and topped with sliced strawberries, peaches, blueberries, and walnuts makes for a tasty, light snack or dessert.

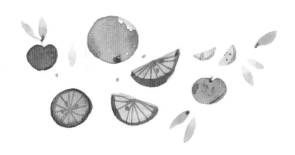

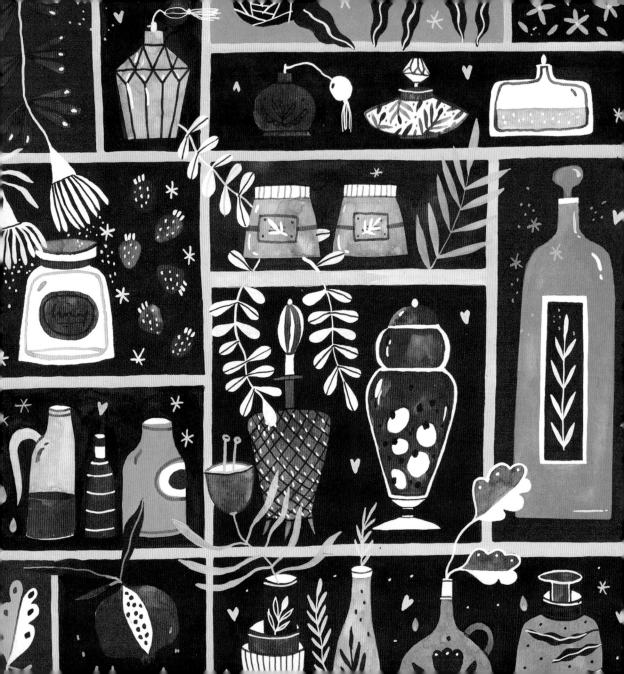

CHAPTER 8

Aphrodite's Apothecary
Everything You Need

THIS COMPREHENSIVE LISTING of ingredients takes you on a journey through the realm of homemade herbal products. Use this compendium as a reference as you create your own love potions.

If this is your first foray into making herbal products, you may find your head spinning as you flip through the pages of ingredients. "Where the heck do I find this stuff?" you might wonder. Don't worry; most of these ingredients are quite readily available. Your local health food store, food co-op, or whole foods grocer is the first place to check. The Internet, of course, is a go-to resource for just about everything you'll need to create all the recipes in this book. I purchase from mail-order catalogs or Internet sources that I know and trust. I prefer sources that I know have a relatively rapid turnover of stock, so I can be sure the ingredients I purchase are fresh. (For a listing of my trusted suppliers, see the resources, page 164.)

Base Oils

Base oils are chemically classified as fats — they contain fatty acids and glycerin — and are derived from beans, nuts, seeds, fruits, flowers, and grains. You may also hear them called unctuous oils, fixed oils, vegetable oils, or carrier oils. Base oils are characteristically greasy, slippery, smooth in texture, and lighter than water, with an extremely low evaporation rate.

Base oils, as their name implies, are used as a base or carrying agent to which essential oils, solid fats, herbs, or spices are added to make herb-infused oils, butters and balms, bath and massage oils, perfume oils, and so on. Base oils can also be used singly or in combination to create massage and skin-conditioning oils. I use only pure, plant-derived oils, never lanolin, lard, cod liver oil, or mineral oil, as I find plant oils to be completely biocompatible with the skin, triggering very few skin sensitivities and having no objectionable odors.

A wonderful benefit to using base oils in body-care and aphrodisiac products is that as they are absorbed, they leave a protective, skin-conditioning barrier on the surface while delivering the herbal benefits to the tissues beneath.

CHOOSING A BASE OIL

The best base oils are those that have been organically grown, naturally extracted, and minimally processed. Look on the label for the key words *organic*, *cold pressed* or *expeller pressed*, or *unrefined* — these guarantee the highest quality. These oils have not been exposed to extraction procedures using petroleum-derived solvents such as hexane (the most common), nor to extremely high temperatures, bleaching, or deodorizing. These processes can destroy or alter an oil's natural molecular state, thereby affecting aromas, flavors, colors, consistency, antioxidant properties, and vitamin, mineral, and essential fatty acid content.

It's important to note that most unrefined base oils — with the exception of avocado, coconut, extra-virgin olive, jojoba, and sesame — have a relatively short shelf life and tend to become rancid if stored at room temperature for more than 8 months, especially in warm weather. These oils should be refrigerated and used, ideally, within 1 year. If an oil you purchase has a strange or "off" smell (note that sesame, coconut, and extra-virgin olive naturally have strong fragrances), then it's probably rancid and should

be returned to where you bought it. Purchase base oils through reputable retailers with a high turnover of inventory, and always check the expiration date on the bottle.

Each base oil used in my recipes has individual characteristics such as texture, weight, slip (how it glides or flows onto the skin), fragrance, ability to penetrate the skin, shelf life, and so on, which determine how it is blended and its intended purpose. There is indeed a method to my madness! Kitchen chemistry is a fun art learned over time, and I encourage you to explore its many facets.

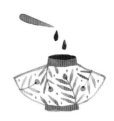

Almond Oil, Sweet

Derived from the ripened, pressed kernel, this is an all-purpose, pale golden, nutritious, very emollient, light- to medium-weight oil with a neutral to slightly warming energy. It has a high fatty acid content that penetrates and reconditions the skin. It is recommended for all skin types, especially dry, inflamed, or itchy skin.

Possible substitute: Apricot kernel oil

Apricot Kernel Oil

Derived from the kernel of the apricot, this oil has properties similar to almond oil, though it's a bit lighter in weight and texture and slightly astringent. A balancing oil that penetrates readily, it gives the skin a lustrous appearance.

Apricot kernel oil has an exquisite fruity aroma (if you purchase unrefined, organic oil) that is not to be missed, and it is excellent for sensitive skin, including mature skin.

Possible substitute: Almond oil

Avocado Oil

Derived primarily from the flesh of the fruit, this full-bodied, medium- to dark-green oil has a gently warming energy and is rich in nutritive and skin-conditioning components such as vitamins A, B1, B2, D, and E; amino acids; lecithin; and essential fatty acids that are especially beneficial to very dry, chapped, irritated, or mature skin.

Because of its medium to slightly heavy emollient texture, this oil takes a bit longer than other base oils to penetrate the top layer of the skin. I always blend it with a lighter oil such as almond or sunflower seed.

Possible substitute: Sesame seed or extra-virgin olive oil, but be aware that they are a bit heavier, and their aromas are quite distinctive.

Castor Oil

This clear to slightly amber-gold, shiny, viscous oil is processed from castor beans. It's highly emollient and analgesic and has a warming energy. Castor oil is the primary oil in most creamy and glossy lipsticks on the commercial market, and it provides staying power and shine to natural lip balm and gloss recipes.

Coconut Oil

Use only organic, extra-virgin, unrefined coconut oil. Its sweet, exotic fragrance and smooth flavor are reminiscent of a tropical paradise (whereas refined coconut oil is devoid of both fragrance and flavor). Coconut oil is derived from the fruit of the coconut palm and is solid at temperatures below 76°F, so in cooler climates it will also act as a natural thickening agent in the recipe to which it is added.

Highly emollient and absorbable, with superior skin-softening properties, it's an excellent oil for all-over use. This tasty, anti-inflammatory, energetically cooling oil also makes the perfect chemical-free intimate lubricant.

Caution: Coconut oil is not latex-friendly.

Jojoba Oil

This light- to medium-weight oil (technically a liquid wax ester) is derived from the seeds of a desert shrub. Chemically similar to our own moisturizing sebum, with a neutral to slightly warm energy, jojoba oil has natural antioxidant and anti-inflammatory properties and penetrates extremely well, leaving no oily residue. Makes skin feel like velvet!

It is one of my favorite oils for making bath and body oils and natural oil-based perfumes because it does not turn rancid and requires no refrigeration.

Olive Oil, Extra Virgin

Derived from the first pressing of ripe olives, this rich, green, relatively stable, moderately heavy oil has a rather strong aroma and taste, so if you choose to use it in formulations, keep in mind that it can dominate other scents and flavors. It contains high levels of monounsaturated fatty acids, antioxidants, enzymes, vitamins, and minerals. In formulations it can be used alone or blended with lighter, less aromatic oils.

With its neutral energy, highly emollient quality, and gently antiseptic and stimulant properties, olive oil is wonderful for use in the bath and as a massage or conditioning body oil. Dry skin drinks it up!

Possible substitutes: Avocado, jojoba, and sesame oils

Sesame Seed Oil

Pressed from sesame seeds, this medium to moderately heavy, light gold, antioxidant oil is rich in vitamins A and E, minerals, and protein and has a slightly warming energy. It has a distinct aroma and taste, so if you choose to use it in formulations, keep in mind that it can dominate other scents and flavors.

Traditionally used in Ayurvedic medicine as a highly emollient massage oil to nourish, condition, and protect the skin from the sun's harmful rays, it can also calm a nervous, anxious disposition, so it's perfect to use on yourself or your partner at the end of a long, stressful day to help you relax and unwind.

Sunflower Oil

Derived from the pressed seeds, this light- to medium-weight oil is rich in essential fatty acids, lecithin, proteins, minerals, and vitamins A and E. Deeply nourishing and moisturizing with a slightly sweet flavor and cooling energy, it is an all-purpose, inexpensive oil.

Possible substitute: Almond oil

Vitamin E Oil

This antioxidant oil, commonly derived from soy or sunflower sources, acts as both a healing agent in personal lubricants as well as a natural preservative in oil-based recipes such as bath and massage oils and oil-based perfumes. I generally call for 1,000 IU of liquid vitamin E oil for every cup (8 ounces) of base oil. Using 500 IU or larger capsules is most convenient; simply pierce the capsules and squeeze out the oil. Buy organic, if available, as most natural vitamin E oils are extracted from genetically modified plants.

Essential Oils

If you have ever enjoyed the heady scent of a rose blossom, the pungency of a fresh peppermint leaf crushed in your hand, the sweet and spicy fragrance of ground cinnamon wafting through the kitchen while baking a batch of cookies, or the light and bright essence that oozes from an orange when you remove its rind, then you've experienced the aromatic qualities of essential oils.

These highly concentrated, intensely aromatic chemical compounds give plants their distinctive smells, but they also play a vital role in plant biochemistry, allowing them to attract pollinators, repel pests, and communicate with nearby plants. They are extracted from plants primarily through careful steam distillation, though there are other methods, such as supercritical carbon dioxide (CO_2) and solvent extraction.

Citrus oils are generally cold-pressed from the fruit's rind.

Essential oils are usually liquid but can be quite viscous (as is the case for Australian sandalwood, ylang-ylang, vetiver, vanilla CO_2, jasmine sambac absolute, and patchouli), semisolid (as for peppermint and rose, depending on the temperature), or even solid (such as orris root). To measure out one of these thicker essential oils from its bottle, just set the bottle in a shallow bowl of warm water, or wrap it with a dark cloth and set it in the sun for a few minutes so it dissolves into a liquid. Then you will be able to dispense it with a sterile glass dropper or an attached drop-by-drop reducer cap, which is how most essential oil bottles under 2 ounces are sealed.

Unlike base oils, essential oils are not actually "oils" because they do not contain fatty acids and are not prone to rancidity, and because of their minute molecular makeup, they evaporate easily (hence their other common name, volatile oils). They react with water much as fatty oils do, by floating to the surface. They do, however, readily lend their scent to water and watery solutions such as hydrosols and vinegar, blend quite readily with base oils and other fats, and dissolve in pure ethyl alcohol, making them an ideal formulary ingredient. In this book

How to Do an Essential Oil Patch Test

Combine 1 or 2 drops of the essential oil in question with ½ teaspoon of base oil in a tiny bowl. Apply a dab on your wrist, inside your upper arm, behind your ear, or behind your knee, and wait 12 to 24 hours. If no irritation develops, it is generally safe to use the essential oil.

their primary use is as an enticing fragrance or flavor additive in the creation of bath and massage oils, body powders, balms, perfumes, and other preparations.

HOW DO ESSENTIAL OILS AFFECT THE BODY?

An essential oil can contain millions of molecules (some of which are quite fragrant and others not so much). These tiny molecules rapidly penetrate the skin, whether applied neat (undiluted) or diluted in a carrier oil, and the vapors easily penetrate the mucous membranes of the respiratory system when inhaled. The molecules then travel quickly through the capillaries and into the circulatory system, which transports them around the body.

As the complex array of molecules travel through the body, they interact with the body's own chemistry, exerting therapeutic effects — sometimes profoundly so — and initiating various

ESSENTIAL OIL SAFETY TIPS

Essential oils are highly concentrated forms of herbal chemical energy, and they must be used with respect and caution. Only some essential oils may be used neat (undiluted) on the skin, those generally being lavender, Peru balsam, geranium (rose geranium), neroli, petitgrain, rose, jasmine, cedarwood, cardamom, frankincense (CO_2), myrrh, patchouli, Australian sandalwood, ylang-ylang, vetiver, and vanilla (CO_2), plus a few other oils used primarily for medicinal purposes. (And even though these are considered some of the safest essential oils, they should still be used sparingly and as directed.)

Always dilute an essential oil in a base oil unless you know it's safe to use neat. It's important to educate yourself about the properties of each essential oil before you use it. The National Association for Holistic Aromatherapy (www.naha.org) — of which I'm a professional member — maintains a website with myriad resources for the essential oil enthusiast. I highly recommend it!

If you rub or splash an essential oil into your nose or eyes — which can cause excruciating pain — immediately flush the affected area with an unscented, bland fatty oil such as olive, almond, sunflower, or generic vegetable. Full-fat cream, half-and-half, or whole milk makes an acceptable substitute for the fatty oil in an emergency. Using plain water does not help; essential oils are attracted to fats alone. Should the pain continue or should severe headache or respiratory irritation develop, seek prompt medical attention, and take the essential oil bottle with you so the attending medical staff knows what they are dealing with.

physiological and psychological functions, such as relief from pain, healing of damaged skin tissue, stimulation or relaxation of the senses, release of hormones, heightening or lessening of libido, enhancement of sexual attraction, or a positive boost in mood or cognitive ability.

Additionally, through our sense of smell, the aromatic vapors stimulate the olfactory nerve — the only nerve in the body that is in direct contact with the external environment — and transmit odor signals directly to the limbic system of the brain. This is the same area of the brain that houses and triggers memories, emotions, desires,

and appetites. Is it any wonder that scent can be such a powerful factor in romantic attraction and desire?

STORING ESSENTIAL OILS

Essential oils retain their healing properties for several years if properly stored in a dark, dry, cool place, and some actually improve with age. The exceptions to this are citrus, pine, and fir oils: They will remain potent for only 6 to 12 months unless refrigerated. When refrigerated, they may last for up to 2 years if not opened frequently.

To prolong the shelf life of an essential oil, do not store the oil in a bottle with a rubber dropper top. The strong vapors emitting from the oil will gradually weaken the rubber, allowing air to enter the bottle, and the precious volatile healing properties will evaporate prematurely. All essential oil bottles should be sealed

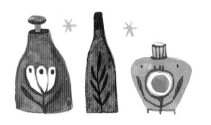

with a plastic screw-top cap, tightly closed at all times. For dispensing, use a sterile glass dropper, though, most oils in bottle sizes under 1 ounce come with drop-by-drop "reducers" for easy application.

If you would like to learn more about purchasing and using high-quality essential oils, I recommend that you educate yourself by reading a couple of good books on the topic and taking a local aromatherapy class, if one is available. I also recommend that you call the company whose oils you want to use and talk to someone in the know about the origins of their oils and production methods used. I purchase my essential oils from a handful of companies I've come to know and trust (see the resources, page 164).

CHOOSING AN ESSENTIAL OIL

On the following pages you'll find a listing of all the essential oils called for in the recipes in this book. But our sense of smell — our sense of what smells good, bad, alluring, repellent, comforting, or arousing — is unique to the individual, so I encourage you to play around with the formulas to find what you like best. The descriptions here focus on each essential oil's fragrance profile and how it can promote well-being, enhance the celebration of romance, or heighten feelings of sensuality, but many of these oils have potent medicinal properties as well. If you want to learn more about their healing effects, turn to the resources on page 164.

Allspice
(Pimenta dioica, P. officinalis)

The allspice berry, with its uplifting, spicy, sweet, warm scent, is so called because it smells and tastes like a combination of juniper berries, cinnamon, black pepper, and cloves. The essential oil is used extensively as an aromatic component in cosmetics and perfumes.

Contraindications: Avoid in pregnancy or epilepsy. Use in moderation and always highly diluted; may be a potential skin irritant.

Balsam Fir
(Abies balsamea)

With a scent reminiscent of a freshly cut Christmas tree, balsam fir essential oil is produced from the tree's needles. Its stimulating scent is superfresh, softly sweet, warming, and almost fruity — fabulous stuff!

Upon deep inhalation, it will definitely open your respiratory channels — it's like a walk through an evergreen forest! Some people find the aroma energizing, though others find it deeply relaxing and quite grounding.

Contraindications: Avoid in pregnancy or epilepsy. May be a potential skin irritant.

Bay Laurel
(Laurus nobilis)

Steam-distilled from the dried leaves of this popular culinary herb, bay has a strong, stimulating, spicy, almost medicinal scent. It frequently makes an appearance in traditional English lavender colognes and perfume oils — which is how I use it.

Contraindications: Avoid in pregnancy or epilepsy. May be a potential skin irritant.

Bergamot
(Citrus bergamia)

Produced by cold expression of the peel of the nearly ripe fruit, which looks much like a miniature orange, the scent is a sweet-fruity-floral citrus with a slightly spicy-balsamic undertone. It has refreshing, mentally uplifting, relaxing qualities and a heating energy. Bergamot oil is what gives Earl Grey tea its lovely flavor and aroma.

Contraindications: Avoid in pregnancy or epilepsy. Use in moderation and highly diluted; may be photosensitizing and a potential skin irritant.

Black Pepper
(Piper nigrum)

With a fresh, dry-woody, warm, spicy scent, along with stimulant properties and a heating energy, black pepper essential oil is produced from dried unripe black peppercorns. When used in very small quantities, it makes an interesting addition to perfume blends and is considered an aphrodisiac.

Contraindications: Avoid in pregnancy or epilepsy. Use in moderation and highly diluted; may be a potential skin irritant.

Cardamom
(Elettaria cardamomum)

Distilled from the seeds of the dried ripe fruit, cardamom has a soft, sweet, spicy scent with woody-citrus undertones. It is warming and gently stimulating to the body, and especially the emotions.

Cedarwood, Virginia
(Juniperus virginiana)

This essential oil, derived from the tree's wood, has the scent that we associate with cedar chests — a fresh, woodsy-sweet, somewhat balsamic, stimulating evergreen fragrance.

Contraindications: Avoid if pregnant.

Chamomile, Roman
(Chamaemelum nobile, Anthemis nobilis)

This golden essential oil, distilled from the small, daisy-like flowers of this delicate, creeping herb, has a sweet, herbaceous, apple-like fragrance with a cooling to neutral energy. It has soothing, calming, anti-inflammatory, nervine properties that help relieve emotional anxiety and physical tension.

Combine it with sweet marjoram and cardamom essential oils to make a softly aromatic, relaxing massage oil blend to ease stress and muscle aches (for the recipe, see page 70).

Cinnamon Bark
(Cinnamomum zeylanicum, C. verum)

With a deep, sweet, spicy, familiar and comforting aroma, the essential oil derived from the dried inner bark of the cinnamon tree adds zip and heat to any blend and is a circulatory-stimulating aphrodisiac. Make sure your cinnamon essential oil is sweetly scented, not acidic or harsh, or it will dominate and ruin the blend. If in doubt, you may substitute a good-quality cinnamon flavoring oil in your recipes, adding and blending 1 drop at a time.

Contraindications: Avoid in pregnancy or epilepsy. Use in moderation and highly diluted; may be photosensitizing and a potential skin irritant.

Clary Sage
(Salvia sclarea)

Distilled from the flowering tops and leaves of this perennial herb, this oil has a tenacious and unusual pungent, sweet, nutty-musky, herbaceous scent, with calming, uplifting, and aphrodisiac effects and a neutral to warming energy. This is especially an oil for women, as it delivers a sense of empowerment and clarity, eases psychological tension, and helps balance hormones.

Contraindications: Avoid in pregnancy or epilepsy.

Clove
(Syzygium aromaticum, syn. Eugenia caryophyllata)

One of the oldest essential oils, familiar and aromatic clove oil has a sweet, spicy, pungent, almost sharp odor with a peculiar fruity-fresh top note. It is steam-distilled from the plant's buds. Like cinnamon bark, this essential oil adds zip and heat to any blend and is a circulatory-stimulating aphrodisiac.

Contraindications: Avoid in pregnancy or epilepsy. Use in moderation and highly diluted, as it is a potential skin irritant.

Frankincense CO_2
(Boswellia carterii)

The CO_2 stands for "supercritical carbon dioxide extraction," and I prefer this type of extraction of the frankincense tree exudates (oleo gum resins) over the steam-distilled version — it's richer, smoother, and sweeter. The fragrance of frankincense is heating, pungent, complex, and strongly diffusive, with hints of fresh terpene and an almost green, lemon-like pepperiness, followed by a rich sweet-balsamic-woody undertone.

Among its properties is the ability to slow down and deepen the breath and preserve spiritual energy, resulting in a calmer, more meditative, receptive mind.

Geranium, Rose
(Pelargonium graveolens)

Most often you'll find this essential oil listed as simply "geranium." It is derived from the leaves, stalks, and flowers of the scented geranium, not the common variety, and has a rather tenacious earthy-green, flowery, rose-like scent, with uplifting, centering, gently stimulating, aphrodisiacal properties and a cooling energy.

This oil is a special gift for women because of its effects on menstrual symptoms, being balancing, calming, and antidepressive. The Bourbon variety is preferred in perfumery formulations as its fragrance is sweeter and more rosy than that of its Chinese cousin, but either will work well in my recipes.

Ginger
(Zingiber officinale)

Produced from the root of this familiar spice, ginger essential oil has a softly fresh, woody-spicy scent with a tenacious sweet, heavy, almost balsamic floral undertone. It has a heating energy and grounding, stimulating, and aphrodisiacal properties.

Contraindications: Avoid in pregnancy or epilepsy. Use in moderation and highly diluted; may be a potential skin irritant.

Grapefruit
(Citrus paradisi)

Cold-pressed from the fruit's peel, this light, sweet-tart, refreshing essential oil with a stimulating aroma and warming energy helps balance moods, lift spirits, and boost self-esteem.

Contraindications: Avoid in pregnancy or epilepsy.

Jasmine Sambac, Absolute
(Jasminum sambac)

It takes nearly eight million jasmine blossoms, hand-picked before the heat of the day on the day the flowers open, to produce just over 2 pounds of superior essential oil, so, like rose essential oil, it is one of the most expensive essential oils on the market. Consequently, it is often adulterated for profit, so know your source! The "absolute" that I use is a highly concentrated, dark orange-brown, viscous liquid and has been produced by solvent extraction.

Having a tenacious and powerfully erotic, hypnotic, rich, intensely floral aroma with an herbaceous-sweet, tea-like undertone, it is one of the oldest aphrodisiac fragrances. Jasmine has uplifting, sensory-stimulating effects and a cooling energy and is balancing to both male and female hormones. I use it, and neroli essential oil, by the drop, primarily for scenting my hair. Both are exquisite!

Juniper Berry
(Juniperus communis)

The refreshing, woodsy-sweet, pine-needle-like fragrance of this essential oil, derived from the berries of the common evergreen shrub, is uplifting and stimulating during times of stress and fatigue. It has a heating energy.

Contraindications: Avoid in pregnancy or epilepsy or if you have kidney problems. May be a potential skin irritant.

Lavender
(Lavandula angustifolia)

Steam-distilled from the beautiful, highly aromatic lavender buds, this essential oil has an old-fashioned, softly sweet-herbaceous, floral aroma with a woody-green undertone and is one of the top scents that turn men on. It has a slightly cooling/neutral energy with relaxing, calming, soothing effects.

Lavender is said to balance the central nervous system. It serves as the main aromatic component in classic English lavender colognes and perfumes.

Lemon
(Citrus limon)

Lemon is one of the most common essential oils and is cold pressed from the fruit's peel. It has a familiar light, fresh, sharp, cooling, cleansing aroma. Its uplifting energy serves as a refreshing stimulant to the nervous system.

Contraindications: Avoid in pregnancy or epilepsy. Use in moderation and highly diluted; may be photosensitizing and a potential skin irritant.

Lime, Sweet
(Citrus aurantifolia)

Bittersweet citrus, derived from the pressed peel, is an interesting fragrance addition that's intensely fresh, fruity, sweet, and rich, with a hint of sea salt essence — difficult to describe, but decidedly aphrodisiacal, and absolutely glorious when combined with petitgrain essential oil.

It has a cooling energy that is mentally stimulating to some; others find that it relieves stress and anxiety. If you love citrus and the smell of fresh ocean air, you have to try my recipe for Sea Salt Seduction Solid Perfume on page 47. It's heavy with the essence of lime and guaranteed to get your lover's attention!

Contraindications: Avoid in pregnancy or epilepsy. Use in moderation and highly diluted; may be photosensitizing and a potential skin irritant.

Marjoram, Sweet
(Origanum majorana)

A tasty culinary herb related to oregano, marjoram has a persistent pungent, woody-sweet-camphoraceous aroma reminiscent of cardamom and nutmeg, with a heating energy. It is actually considered an anti-aphrodisiac as it has been used by women wishing to decrease sexual advances by their partners, but this is not the reason I included it in this book.

Because it is quite tranquilizing to the nervous system, and positively wonderful for easing emotional exhaustion, sore muscles, and tension headaches, it makes a great additive to a comforting massage oil blend to use on your partner when you just want to shower him or her with tender, loving care . . . not seduce him or her.

Contraindications: Avoid in pregnancy or epilepsy.

Myrrh
(Commiphora myrrha)

One of the oldest essential oils, it's produced from distillation of certain tree exudates (gum resins) and has a very warm, rich, heavy, slightly medicinal, spicy-balsamic odor with centering, grounding, and gently sedating properties.

It is said to instill awareness and confidence upon the wearer of the oil. Myrrh is also available as a sweeter CO_2 extraction, which I really like.

Contraindications: Avoid in pregnancy or epilepsy.

Neroli
(Citrus aurantium)

Neroli essential oil is distilled from orange blossoms of the bitter orange tree and named after a princess of Nerola in Italy, who wore it as her signature perfume. Traditionally, stems of orange blossoms were used in bridal bouquets to calm nervous apprehension before the couple retired to the marital bed.

Neroli has a rich, powerful yet delicate, hauntingly erotic floral scent, with a sweet-terpeney top note and cooling energy. Intensely fragrant, it is best appreciated in very mild dilutions.

It has a special affinity for women in almost any stage of transition; it eases menstrual cramps, assists in menopause, and is wonderful for anxiety and depression. Having deeply soothing and uplifting effects, neroli has a special place among aphrodisiacs. Like rose and jasmine essential oils, it is on the expensive side, so I use it judiciously, by the drop, primarily for scenting my hair.

Nutmeg
(Myristica fragrans)

Gently stimulating, sensual, and very grounding, nutmeg has a rather potent aroma with a distinctly terpeney top note and a rich, sweet-spicy, warm body note that can easily dominate blends. Used in excess, it can have a dulling sensation on the brain, acting as a sedative.

Contraindications: Avoid in pregnancy or epilepsy. Use in moderation and highly diluted; may be a potential skin irritant.

Orange, Sweet
(Citrus sinensis)

One of the least expensive and most common essential oils produced, sweet orange essential oil is cold-pressed from the ripe rind of the orange fruit. With its familiar fresh, light yet rich, sweet and fruity aroma, and its warming energy, orange oil is beneficial for anxiety, nervousness, and sadness — wonderful for opening the heart, creating a "sunshine" effect that makes you feel good all over. Depending on what you need, it can either help relax or energize your being. It is particularly appealing to men.

Contraindications: Avoid in pregnancy or epilepsy. Use in moderation and highly diluted; may be photosensitizing and a potential skin irritant.

Palmarosa
(Cymbopogon martinii)

A close relative to lemongrass, with a rich, heavy, sweet, rosy-floral fragrance, palmarosa has a cooling, balancing energy and soothing, uplifting, aphrodisiacal properties. I like to blend this with rose absolute and rose geranium essential oils.

Patchouli
(Pogostemon cablin)

A dark amber, viscous oil distilled from the dried, typically fermented leaves, patchouli essential oil has a distinctive, extremely rich, earthy-sweet-herbaceous, spicy-woody-balsamic aroma that deepens and gets better with age (just like we do!).

Warming and calming, it is said to dispel nervous exhaustion and stress-related complaints — lending a "laid-back" effect. Patchouli synthetic fragrance oil is often marketed as "natural," so know your source and be sure you're getting the pure essential oil.

Peppermint
(Mentha piperita)

Derived from the leaves and flowers, peppermint is refreshing, highly aromatic, and pungent, with a powerful minty bite and cooling energy. It's quite stimulating to the respiratory channels; some find it energizing, while others find it rather relaxing.

Contraindications: Avoid in pregnancy or epilepsy.

Peru Balsam
(Myroxylon balsamum var. pereirae)

Produced from the crude balsam of this tropical tree, the essential oil is a pale amber or brown semiviscous liquid with a rich, sweet, heavy, balsamic, vanilla-like scent. It has warming, opening, grounding, and comforting qualities; it soothes tension and stress.

Petitgrain
(Citrus aurantium)

Reminiscent of sweet orange flowers with penetrating spicy, woody-herbaceous undertones, this oil is produced from the leaves, twigs, and unripe fruit of the same tree that produces bitter orange oil and orange blossom oil (neroli).

It has a warming energy with grounding, calming, mentally clarifying, and uplifting properties — absolutely heavenly. It's one of my favorites and, unlike the other citrus oils, is nonirritant, nonsensitizing, and nonphototoxic.

Rose Absolute
(Rosa damascena, R. centifolia)

World renowned as an aphrodisiac, rose essential oil has an exquisite, intoxicating, almost narcotic floral aroma. It is one of the most beloved, most precious, most expensive essential oils on the market. It can take approximately 60 roses to produce just 1 drop of this oil; thus the steep price. It is often adulterated for profit, so know your source!

An absolute, which is what I use in this book, is solvent-extracted from the fresh petals, less costly, and used exclusively as a perfume. The more expensive rose otto is steam-distilled and preferred over the solvent-extracted absolute for aromatherapy work. Rose essential oil has an affinity for the heart, keeping it open and connected to all things. It is uplifting in times of emotional stress, grief, sadness, and depression, yet calming to the nerves.

If you adore roses, you owe it to yourself to purchase a bottle of either rose absolute or rose otto — you're worth it! Better yet, put it on your birthday list — perhaps your lover will indulge your fragrance passion.

Rosemary
(Rosmarinus officinalis chemotype *verbenon)*

Known as "the herb of remembrance," rosemary essential oil is distilled from the fresh flowering tops and resinous leaves and has a strong, sharp, camphoraceous, herbaceous aroma with a warming energy.

I prefer the chemotype verbenon to camphor and cineol for its gentleness on the skin, more citrusy aroma, and slightly relaxing, yet clearing and uplifting effects. Rosemary stimulates memory, creativity, confidence, and mental energy.

Contraindications: Avoid in pregnancy or epilepsy.

Sandalwood, Australian
(Santalum spicatum)

Australian sandalwood is sustainably grown and harvested. This species is used similarly to Indian sandalwood (*Santalum album*), which is endangered. The scent has a woody, musky-balsamic, extremely tenacious base with a light, dry, spicy top note, balanced by a cooling energy and grounding, centering, aphrodisiacal properties. It is useful for relieving tension and anxiety.

Spearmint
(Mentha spicata)

The milder cousin of peppermint, spearmint is lighter, sweeter, and softer with a gently cooling, stimulating energy that refreshes and tingles the senses.

Vanilla CO$_2$
(Vanilla planifolia)

A warming aphrodisiac loved by both men and women, this familiar rich, creamy, sweetly spicy, somewhat woody, tobacco-like, and oh-so-sensual fragrance softens all blends. It is often adulterated and synthesized — know your source!

Vanilla essential oil acts as a relaxant for anger, tension, irritability, and stress, making it the perfect additive for relaxing massage oils. Premium essential oil from "cured" Madagascar vanilla beans is naturally thick, dark brown, and resinous, and it blends especially well with vetiver, spices, mints, resins, and citrus oils.

Vetiver
(Vetiveria zizanioides)

With an earthy-woody, very heavy, exotic aroma, a sweet, persistent undertone, and comforting, relaxing, warming energy, vetiver essential oil comes from the rootlets of this tall, tufted, scented grassy plant. In India and Sri Lanka the essence is known as "the oil of tranquility."

Nothing brings you back to your center as strongly as vetiver. It is reputed to have an aphrodisiac effect for both sexes and to act as a hormone balancer for women.

Ylang-Ylang
(Cananga odorata)

An intensely sweet, tenacious, exquisite fragrance with a floral-woody undertone, exotic hint of spice, and cooling energy, ylang-ylang is steam-distilled from the large, tender flowers of a tropical tree. In Indonesia, where it grows wild, it is customary to spread the flowers on the beds of newly married couples, where its heady scent serves as an alluring aphrodisiac.

Hydrosols

Aromatic hydrosols are typically a natural, watery by-product of the essential oil distillation process, though some superior-quality hydrosols are made by devoted distillers who steam small batches of fresh floral and plant material strictly to produce hydrosol. These aromatic essences have therapeutic properties similar to those of essential oils, but in much lower concentrations, and they contain the water-soluble elements from the distilled plant. Most aromatic sprays or "flower waters" on the market are not pure hydrosols but rather essential oils added to water with an emulsifier. These are chemically different from hydrosols and are not as gentle.

Hydrosols have scents that are generally mild and subtle, but sometimes bright and fragrant, and most have an herby or grassy note. They are packaged in glass or metal spray containers and can be used as hydrating facial spritzers, fragrant hair mists, ultralight body scents, or captivating linen sprays for your boudoir. They must be kept in a cool, dark place and generally have a shelf life of 1 year or less. Here are some of my favorites.

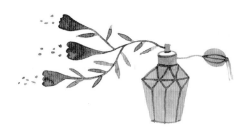

Cucumber
(Cucumis sativus)

Produced from the cucumber fruit, it's very refreshing, crisp, and cooling. It's also one of the scents that women find most alluring.

Geranium, Rose
(Pelargonium graveolens)

Distilled from the aerial plant parts, this essence has a grassy, flowery, and rose-like aroma, with a hint of lemon. With a cooling energy and uplifting, centering, gently stimulating, and aphrodisiacal properties, it's also a great balancer, ideal for hormonal ups and downs, including hot flashes — a precious and valuable hydrosol for women in all stages of life.

Lavender or Lavandin
(Lavandula angustifolia,
L. x intermedia)

This is herbaceous, grassy, and muted, not a sweet floral like lavender buds or lavender essential oil. It relaxes and refreshes the senses with a unique scent that appeals to both men and women.

Lemon Verbena
(Aloysia triphylla)

A lemony-green, slighted muted, light essence distilled from the leaves, this gently stimulating, refreshing, revitalizing scent is like a breath of summer in a bottle. Many find it eases nervous tension and anxiety.

Lime
(Citrus aurantifolia)

This invigorating, cooling, crisp, sweet scent with the essence of sea salt and lime peel reminds me of citrus groves and ocean breezes.

Neroli
(Citrus aurantium)

This is true orange blossom, a rich yet delicate, cooling floral with deeply soothing effects. If you find the essential oil too tenacious, then this lighter version is for you — it's exotic and heavenly.

Rose
(Rosa damascena)

Rose is classically sensuous, adored by most everyone. If you love the scent of rose essential oil but find it a bit overwhelming or rich at times, this might appeal to you. Ever-so-subtle and soft, it opens the heart and soothes emotional upsets.

Herbs & Spices

Each herb and spice has a unique energy and special properties that can enhance your celebrations of romance and sensuality in many ways. Some may help lift your libido or restore vitality, while others serve as tonics that nourish your body and mind or help you adapt to stress. Some stimulate energy, while others relax your being, soothe your senses, and balance your mood. Still others are excellent as flavoring or aroma additives, whether you're making an edible "body dessert" or an alluring perfume. All have something wonderful to offer and are worth exploring.

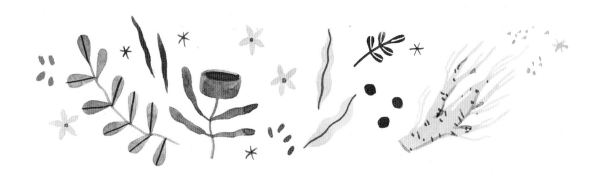

Alkanet
(Alkanna tinctoria)

Also known as dyer's bugloss or Spanish bugloss, alkanet root has been used for centuries as a dye for pharmaceuticals and cosmetics. The thick root releases a stunning blood-red color in oils and waxes, but not in water. I use it to lend coloring to my rose-infused solid perfumes.

Allspice
(Pimenta dioica, P. officinalis)

This common kitchen spice has an uplifting, sweet, warm scent. For a hint of spicy bite, I add a few whole dried berries to my Cherry Kissing Cordial (see the recipe on page 7), and it also makes a nice addition to potpourri blends.

Anise, Star
(Illicium verum)

The seeds of this common Chinese spice, with its intensely sweet licorice-like scent and very warming, pungent flavor, have been used in traditional Chinese medicine for centuries. They are often chewed after meals to sweeten the breath and promote digestion. The whole dried seed-bearing pods are valued as a decorative and fragrant accent in potpourri blends.

Ashwagandha
(Withania somnifera)

Ashwagandha is a shrubby perennial native to the drier subtropical regions of India, Pakistan, Sri Lanka, and Africa. The beige-colored root, with a combination of bitter, astringent, and sweet tastes and a warming energy, is one of the most highly regarded and commonly used adaptogens in the Ayurvedic pharmacopoeia and is often referred to as "Indian ginseng."

It enables the body to reserve and sustain vital energy throughout the day, while promoting sound, restful sleep at night, thereby maximizing the body's ability to manage stress. It is considered one of the best herbs for calming, nourishing, and strengthening an exhausted nervous system.

Its name *ashwagandha*, meaning "the smell of a horse," comes from the odor of the fresh root (like horse's urine), and also perhaps because it is renowned for imparting the vitality and sexual stamina of a horse to both men and women!

Contraindications: Do not use while pregnant or nursing.

Astragalus
(Astragalus membranaceus)

The beige-colored root of this member of the legume family has a sweet taste and gently warming energy. Astragalus is one of the most popular rejuvenating herbs in China and is considered an adaptogenic herb, as it helps the body adapt to change and stress.

It is used to build resistance to disease by strengthening the immune and endocrine systems. Valued as a chi tonic, it increases core energy and overall vitality, improves digestion, and strengthens the lungs, spleen, kidneys, and blood. It is wonderful for those suffering from chronic fatigue.

Calendula
(Calendula officinalis)

Common in most herb gardens — and I strongly suggest planting some seeds if you have room — the sunny orange and yellow calendula flowers, with their neutral to cooling energy, are known for their calming, anti-inflammatory, and vulnerary (wound-healing) properties.

Cardamom
(Elettaria cardamomum)

Cardamom has a soft, sweet, spicy, woody-citrus scent and flavor; it's warming and gently stimulating to the senses when inhaled, yet calming to the digestive system when eaten. This familiar spice is used in liqueur, massage oil, potpourri, and body powder recipes. If you want an amazingly effective breath freshener, chew on a few seeds before you surprise your partner with a big, fat kiss!

Cayenne
(Capsicum annuum)

This vibrantly rust-red pepper has a pungent, hot bite, with drying, circulation-enhancing, stimulating properties. I like to add a pinch of ground cayenne to smoothies and other recipes, as it provides a definite zestiness along with energy-boosting qualities.

Contraindications: Be very careful when handling powdered cayenne, as a mere smidgen can produce a burning sensation if it comes into contact with your eyes, nose, or mouth. Wash your hands immediately after working with this spice.

Chamomile
(Matricaria recutita, M. chamomilla)

The small, daisy-like flowers of this common aromatic herb have a sweet, fresh, herbaceous, apple-like fragrance with a cooling to neutral energy that is most pleasing and relaxing to the senses. It is wonderful for skin that is sensitive or inflamed; I often add a handful of the comforting flowers to herbal bath bag blends. If you have a garden, please plant a patch or two of chamomile; it makes a delicious, calming tea.

Cinnamon
*(Cinnamomum burmannii —
cassia; C. verum — sweet)*

Cinnamon has a familiar, comforting, wonderfully spicy-sweet aroma and flavor. Its heat and stimulating properties enhance energy and boost circulation throughout the body. I use both the powder and the whole "sticks."

Clove
*(Syzygium aromaticum, syn.
Eugenia caryophyllata)*

Cloves offer a pungent, stimulating aroma and flavor in whatever recipe they are added to.

Cocoa, Raw
(Theobroma cacao)

Over 95 percent of the cocoa powder on the market is the end result of the multi-step processing needed to create chocolate liquor, which involves cleaning, fermenting, sorting, roasting, cracking, and grinding of the cacao seed or cocoa bean. Because of the dramatic growth of the raw food movement over the last decade or so, there has been an increased demand for raw cocoa powder (also called cacao powder), made without all that heat.

It is dark, rich, bitter, and amazingly high in health- and beauty-boosting nutrients, plus "feel good" chemical compounds. It's also decadently delicious — I'm a shameless chocoholic, I'll readily admit!

Possible substitutes: If raw cocoa powder or nibs are unavailable, then feel free to use the roasted versions.

Comfrey
(Symphytum officinale)

Comfrey leaf is a "master mender" of all manner of skin irritations; it has mildly astringent, soothing, emollient, conditioning, mucilaginous (slippery and gooey), and vulnerary (wound-healing) properties with a cooling energy.

I blend it with calendula and chamomile flowers to make a gentle, unscented herbal lubricant and massage oil. Comfrey is yet another herb that I recommend growing in your herb garden. She likes to spread out, so give her ample space!

Damiana
(Turnera diffusa, T. aphrodisiaca)

Damiana is an aromatic, low-growing shrubby perennial native to subtropical North America, especially Mexico, California, and Texas. The leaf has a warm energy and a flavor that's slightly bitter/sour, with an astringent aftertaste.

Damiana has a strong reputation as an aphrodisiac, enhancing passion, desire, and romance, and I suspect that it gained this renown because of its potent tonic and restorative properties that aid in bringing relief to symptoms of anxiety, mild depression, impotence, frigidity, and infertility.

Damiana helps increase internal warmth and energy, while delivering a sense of calm, which goes a long way toward restoring sexual vitality and desire.

Eleuthero
(Eleutherococcus senticosus)

This bland-tasting root is imbued with almost magical qualities and has properties and health benefits similar to those of Asian ginseng (*Panax ginseng*). (In fact, it used to be called Siberian ginseng.) Eleuthero root has been traditionally used to stimulate male virility and as a reproductive tonic for men, but it does wonders for women, too.

Highly valued for improving stamina and endurance and boosting circulation, this excellent adaptogenic root, with a gently warming energy, should be taken consistently over time, as it helps restore vitality deep within the tissues, thereby increasing resistance to disease, supporting normal metabolic processes, and enhancing your ability to deal with stress, whether physical, psychological, biological, or environmental. It is also believed to bestow wisdom upon and promote longevity for the consumer.

Possible substitute: American ginseng (Panax quinquefolius) root

Contraindication: Not to be used while pregnant or nursing.

FOR THE LOVE OF CHOCOLATE

Love is the most wonderful of all feelings in this world, isn't it? And the food that most often symbolizes this emotion is chocolate. Now, I'm not talking about the popular Hershey's Kisses or Lindt Lindor Truffles, but real, raw chocolate, also known as cacao. Described as the "food of love" for good reason, cacao contains an abundance of phenylethylamines (PEAs), a class of compounds that we produce in our body when we fall in love. This could be one of the main reasons for the existence of a deep association between chocolate and feelings of love.

Additionally, anandamide, a cannabinoid endorphin that the body naturally produces in the brain after exercise, is also found in cacao. It's known as the "bliss chemical" because it is released while we're feeling wonderful. This natural neurotransmitter is said to stimulate the energy of the heart chakra, stirring feelings of joy, love, bliss, tenderness, affection, and passion.

Both PEAs and anandamide are heat- and alkaline-sensitive; thus, they are only minimally present in cooked (roasted) and processed conventional and organic chocolate. You've got to eat real, raw cacao to truly experience their amazing benefits!

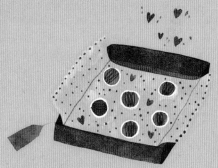

Fo-ti
(Polygonum multiflorum)

Also known as ho sho wu, fo-ti is a renowned classic Chinese rejuvenative, adaptogenic, tonic, and longevity herb, used by millions of people for hundreds of years. This beige- to brown-colored, slightly sweet-tasting root, with a hint of astringent bitterness and gently warming energy, is said to counter the effects of aging, build the blood, increase sperm count in men and promote fertility in women, enhance sexual energy and circulatory function, and strengthen the muscles, ligaments, tendons, and bones.

It helps strengthen yet relax the nervous system — which is why it is a beneficial herb for stress reduction — and build chi, or energy.

Contraindication: Not to be used while pregnant or nursing.

Frankincense
(Boswellia carteri)

This highly aromatic resin is harvested from the tree exudates and was one of the first spices Europeans brought back from the Far East. Frankincense has a heating, pungent, complex, strongly diffusive scent with hints of fresh terpene and an almost green and lemon-like pepperiness, followed by a rich sweet-balsamic-woody undertone. Frankincense "tears" — small pieces of resin — are often used in potpourri and incense blends.

Ginger
(Zingiber officinale)

A familiar gnarly root or rhizome with a fresh, delicious, zippy bite, ginger increases circulation and core energy and is a remarkable healing spice to consume when suffering from indigestion. It has a warm to hot energy and grounding, centering, stimulating, aphrodisiacal properties.

Need a quick breath freshener? Munch on a tiny piece of fresh gingerroot — it's sure to leave your mouth feeling clean, spicy, and oh-so-kissable!

Contraindications: Avoid consumption in cases of stomach inflammation/ulcers or serious digestive or liver problems.

Ginseng, American
(Panax quinquefolius)

I'm a big fan of American ginseng and often combine it with schisandra berries to make a luscious, rejuvenating tonic wine (see my recipe on page 104). American ginseng is considered the best ginseng variety in the world. Though used similarly to Asian ginseng (*Panax ginseng*), it differs in chemical energetics and makeup.

While Asian ginseng is a sweet, slightly bitter, warming stimulant that builds energy and heat in the body, American ginseng is sweet, bitter, and neutral — more soothing, cooling, and less stimulating — making it a better choice for many Americans, who are exhausted, overly stressed, and suffering from mental fog and sexual inadequacy. It has the same adaptogenic and balancing tonic effects as the Asian variety with a long history as a building and restorative herb.

At-risk warning: Suffering from overharvesting and habitat destruction, wild American ginseng is considered at risk or endangered in most of its native growing areas. Use only organically cultivated or woods-grown ginseng (ginseng that has been planted and tended in woodland settings), and always verify the source of your roots.

Possible substitute: Eleuthero (Eleutherococcus senticosus) root

Contraindication: Not to be used while pregnant or nursing.

Hibiscus
(Hibiscus sabdariffa)

This tropical plant with large, deep, vibrant red flowers is commonly available as a houseplant. When dried, the flowers are used for making a stunning red tea that's high in bioflavonoids and vitamin C with a sweet-tart, slightly astringent taste and cooling energy. This is the flower that put Celestial Seasonings teas on the map, and they've used it as a tasty base, colorant, and flavoring ingredient in their blends for decades, as do I.

Kava Kava
(Piper methysticum)

Growing wild in the South Pacific islands, kava is a tall shrub that belongs to the pepper family. Its highly revered root, with a pungent, slightly bitter taste and warming energy, has been used in native folk remedies and ceremonial beverages for hundreds of years for its unique properties, which produce a sense of relaxation and compassion, while allowing you to feel quite aware and alert. Kava is wonderful if you tend to be a nervous sort, as it aids in the reduction of stress and tension.

When you buy kava root powder, taste a smidge; it has a unique flavor, and you'll soon feel a temporary numbing and tingling sensation on your tongue that quickly spreads throughout your mouth — this is due to the active chemical compounds called kavalactones.

Contraindication: Kava is a powerful herb that deserves much respect. Though it has wonderful properties, avoid it if you are pregnant or nursing or have liver problems; if you are taking Coumadin (warfarin) or any other drug that influences blood clotting; if you are taking medications for anxiety or insomnia, as it may enhance drowsiness; or if you are taking antipsychotic drugs or any other medications that influence dopamine levels. If used in excess, kava may make you feel intoxicated, sleepy, or nauseated or may impair your ability to drive or operate heavy machinery. It is not recommended for consumption with alcoholic beverages.

Lavender
(Lavandula angustifolia)

An old-fashioned, romantic flower with a soft, sweet-herbaceous aroma and woody-green undertone, lavender lends a soothing, relaxing fragrance to body-care and bath products. The floral fragrance is a favorite of most women, but men find it especially captivating! A must-grow flower if you have a garden — I always harvest plenty from my plants each summer.

Lemon Balm
(Melissa officinalis)

Lemon balm, also known as melissa, is a bushy perennial, a member of the mint family, and a must-have in your aromatic herb garden. It has a heady, tart, citrus-like, fresh top note with a sweet herbaceous odor and flavor. Lemon balm's main property is as a nervine — it's very calming to the nervous system. Like lemongrass, it adds a tasty flavor and cooling energy to herb tea blends.

Much of the flavor and scent are lost in drying, so use fresh leaves whenever possible. Sixteenth-century herbalist John Gerard declared that it "maketh the heart merry, joyful, strengtheneth the vitall spirits."

Lemongrass
(Cymbopogon citratus)

This grassy plant, native to India and Pakistan and now cultivated in Africa, Indonesia, South America, and China, has a distinctive slightly bitter, pungent, tenacious fragrance and flavor and adds a tasty flavor and cooling energy to herbal tea blends.

Maca
(Lepidium meyenii or L. peruvianum)

Also known as Peruvian ginseng, maca root is considered a powerful adaptogenic herb, which means that it increases the power of resistance against multiple stressors — physical, emotional, biological, or chemical — while also restoring balance and supporting normal metabolic processes. The root, which resembles a young turnip, is rich in many vitamins and minerals, and it has a slightly malty flavor and warming energy.

Maca is a member of the cruciferous family and has been cultivated and grown high in the Peruvian Andes of South America for two thousand years. It is prized for enhancing physical strength, endurance, and libido, as well as balancing moods, supporting healthy hormone production, and increasing energy.

Myrrh
(Commiphora myrrha)

The aromatic gum resin is harvested from the tree exudates and has a warm, heavy, slightly medicinal, spicy-balsamic odor with centering, grounding, and gently sedating properties. As with frankincense, the whole and crushed resin pieces are often used as a fragrance fixative in potpourri and incense blends.

Nutmeg
(Myristica fragrans)

Nutmeg is a very warm, gently stimulating, rather sensual spice with a potent aroma that can easily dominate a recipe if you are heavy-handed. I like to use it as a flavoring in foods and as a fragrance additive in body powders and potpourri.

Peppermint
(Mentha piperita)

I grow a variety of peppermint in my garden called narrow-leaf peppermint or "white" mint (*M. piperita* f. *pallescens*), which is extremely cooling, pungent, and aromatic. Chewing a fresh leaf creates an almost icy taste sensation that's simply out of this world. All peppermint leaves have a powerful, ultrarefreshing bite, so if you have access to a fresh plant, share a leaf with your sweetie. Chew it up, feel the chill, and enjoy a stimulating, minty kiss! Mmmm . . . nice!

Possible substitute: Spearmint leaf

Rose
(Rosa species)

Our beloved roses impart an Old-World, softly sensual, deep, slightly spicy-sweet, floral aroma and cooling energy to all manner of body care and edible recipes. Both the petals and the hips are used.

Saw Palmetto
(Serenoa repens)

A traditional herb long used by the native inhabitants of the coastal plains of the southern United States, this low-growing shrubby palm is valued for its succulent fruit. The dried berries are deep purple; they yield a reddish-brown granular powder with a fatty, pungent, sweet flavor that is rather unpleasant but can be disguised with other herbs.

Saw palmetto berries have a tonic diuretic and relaxant action and can be taken regularly to strengthen the endocrine and urinary systems and to prevent future problems with the prostate gland. In fact, this herb is one of the best remedies for inflammation of the prostate.

This oil- and nutrient-rich fruit is one of the few Western herbs that has anabolic properties: it strengthens and builds body tissue, encouraging weight gain and bulk. Saw palmetto is also recommended for those who tend to be nervous, stressed, and exhausted, as it aids in restoring energy and vitality.

Note: When purchasing the powder, be sure it is of superior quality and very fresh, as the fatty acids contained within quickly turn rancid. Store it, tightly sealed, in the refrigerator to preserve freshness; it will keep for up to 6 months.

Schisandra
(Schisandra chinensis)

Though it is native to northern China and parts of Russia, this deciduous climbing vine with its bright red berries can be grown in North America. Its common Chinese name, *wu wei zi*, means "five-flavored berry," as this spectacular berry, when chewed, releases a flavor explosion of sweet, sour, salty, pungent, and bitter.

Schisandra is an adaptogen, meaning it helps increase resistance to the damaging effects of disease and stress, restores balance, and supports normal metabolic processes. As a harmonizing tonic herb, it serves as an aid to boosting energy, stamina, endurance, and sex drive; normalizing blood sugar and blood pressure; treating liver, lung, kidney, and heart disease; and promoting longevity. Among female herbalists, it has a valued reputation as a preserver of beauty and youthful vitality and as a potent sexual tonic.

Shatavari
(Asparagus racemosus)

A member of the lily family, shatavari root is a primary herb in traditional Ayurvedic herbal medicine for gynecological purposes: to strengthen female hormones, promote fertility, nourish and soothe the female reproductive system, increase production of breast milk, and relieve menstrual pain. For the male reproductive system, it is recommended for use in cases of low sperm count.

The root has a sweet, slightly bitter taste, with a cooling energy. It is also valued for its demulcent property, in that it increases lubrication and moisture where there is inflammation from dryness and heat, plus it enhances physical strength, maintains youthfulness, improves memory, and serves as an adaptogen, helping the body adapt to stressors of all kinds. Shatavari is said to calm the mind and increase love, devotion, and compassion . . . nice attributes!

Shatavari Has an Interesting Meaning

The name *shatavari* can mean "one hundred roots" but is more commonly said to mean "she who has one hundred husbands." It has been used for millennia as an aphrodisiac and to enhance fertility in both women and men. The fresh juice of the plant's roots is used in several classic Ayurvedic formulas claimed to be sexual tonics.

Spearmint
(Mentha spicata)

Lighter, sweeter, and softer, with a gently cooling, stimulating energy that refreshes and tingles the senses, spearmint is the milder cousin of peppermint, and it can be used interchangeably in recipes calling for peppermint.

   If you love mints, plant a few varieties on the outer edges of your garden (they're invasive). By themselves they make great tea, and they are flavorful additions to all kinds of other beverages.

Possible substitute: Peppermint leaf

Vanilla
(Vanilla planifolia)

Smooth, smoldering, deep, rich, sweet, and creamy . . . oh my! The familiar scent of vanilla appeals to just about everyone. If you're a lover of all things vanilla, as I am, you will want to use this aromatic, alluring, luscious bean in as many forms and in as many scentsationally sensual products as possible!

   I use the whole beans when making vanilla-infused massage oil and in my homemade extract (see page 31); the ground vanilla beans as an additive to body powder formulations; the sweetened bean paste to flavor and scent edible body treats; and the extract as a flavoring for food, as well as a body perfume and boudoir fragrance spray.

Thickeners

When making lip balms and glosses, solid perfumes, personal lubricants, and edible body butters and balms at home, natural thickening agents are necessary to give the product its desired density, which can range from a thin lotion-like consistency to a very thick, semihard paste wax. The following ingredients are commonly used by herbalists and kitchen cosmetologists to soothe and moisturize the skin, enhance flavor and fragrance, and help bind the recipe ingredients together.

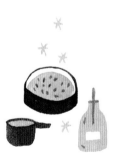

Beeswax

Secreted by worker honeybees, pure, unrefined, unbleached beeswax adds a sweet, honey-like fragrance and golden color to products, and when melted, it hardens quickly as it cools. Beeswax is available in many forms: honeycomb sheets that can be broken or cut; convenient pastilles or pellets that can be measured and melted with ease; or solid blocks and small chunks that can be placed in a ziplock freezer bag and whacked with a hammer to break up into small, measurable pieces.

Possible substitute: Refined vegetable emulsifying wax does not have the same alluring qualities as beeswax but is a good vegan substitute. I prefer to use fresh beeswax, as I appreciate the skin-conditioning properties and adore the aroma.

Cocoa Butter

Derived from the cocoa bean (*Theobroma cacao*), this rich, golden, emollient vegetable fat smells and tastes of chocolate. It is hard at room temperature but melts at body temperature and lends a thick, creamy consistency with gentle, soothing, conditioning properties for the skin. It's a wonderful addition to recipes for personal lubricants, tasty lip balms, and edible body butters.

Caution: Cocoa butter is not latex-friendly.

Ghee

Ghee, an integral part of traditional Indian cuisine, is clarified butter, which means that the water and milk solids (mostly proteins) have been simmered off, leaving just the rich, golden butterfat or oil, which is excellent for cooking. It is shelf stable, never needs refrigeration, and is lactose- and casein-free, so if you are intolerant to butter, try ghee.

In India it is also rubbed into the skin for nourishment. It makes an excellent conditioning oil for an erotic massage and is especially yummy as an "edible body butter" when mixed with raw honey, maple syrup, or a smidge of vegetable glycerin and a drop of sweet orange essential oil.

Caution: Ghee is not latex-friendly.

Glycerin, Vegetable

A natural emollient derived from vegetable fats, this clear, slippery, superthick, moisturizing, water-soluble liquid acts as a humectant (drawing moisture from the air to the skin), but it also pulls moisture from within the skin toward its surface.

If you put a bit on your tongue, you'll notice it has a very sweet, warm taste. I occasionally add it in lieu of honey to lip balms and edible body treats for its sweet flavor and moisturizing quality, and I use it in personal lubricants to help keep sensitive intimate tissues moist and comfortable.

Shea Butter

Pressed from the nuts of the karite tree (*Butyrospermum parkii*), unrefined shea butter, creamy to pale gold in color, is a soft, solid fat, often with a distinct fragrance that's difficult to mask. If the scent displeases you, purchase the refined butter, which is slightly firmer, whiter in color, and much less aromatic. Shea butter contributes a thick, creamy consistency with emollient, skin-softening properties when added to lip and body balms. It can even be used alone.

Shea butter takes much longer to harden than beeswax, so keep that in mind if you decide to use it as the primary thickening ingredient when creating your own recipes.

Resources

Suppliers

ABSOLUTE AROMAS
+44-0-142-054-0400
absolute-aromas.com

AMPHORA AROMATICS
+44-0-117-904-7212
amphora-aromatics.com

THE ANANDA APOTHECARY
888-758-6360
anandaapothecary.com
Therapeutic-grade essential oils and blends, hydrosols, aromatherapy supplies, carrier oils, bottles, essential oil diffusers, and books

AROMATHERAPEUTIX
800-308-6284
aromatherapeutix.com
Essential oils and oil blends, bottles, soaps, herbal body and health care products, essential oil diffusers, and more

THE AROMATHERAPY SHOP
+44-0-203-189-1940
thearomatherapyshop.co.uk

AROMATICS INTERNATIONAL
406-273-9833
aromatics.com
Organic and wildcrafted essential oils and oil blends, hydrosols, carrier oils, essential oil accessories and kits, and packaging

AURA CACIA
Frontier Natural Products Co-op
800-437-3301
auracacia.com
Essential oils, base oils, and natural skin and body care products

AUSTRALIAN BOTANICAL PRODUCTS
+61-03-9709-4800
abp.com.au

AVENA BOTANICALS
866-282-8362
avenabotanicals.com
Organic elixirs, tinctures, glycerites, herbal teas, bulk herbs, natural skin and body care products, books, and more

BANYAN BOTANICALS
800-953-6424
banyanbotanicals.com
Sustainably sourced, certified organic Ayurvedic herbs such as shatavari and ashwagandha, plus other health and body care products for the Ayurvedic lifestyle

BULK APOTHECARY
888-728-7612
bulkapothecary.com
Essential oils, soap and candle making supplies, fragrances and flavorings, herbs and spices, base oils, cosmetic clays, waxes and butters, and more

CAPE BOTTLE CO.
888-833-6307
capebottle.com
Glass, plastic, and tin packaging

CHAMPLAIN VALLEY APIARIES
800-841-7334
champlainvalleyhoney.com
Fresh beeswax, beeswax candles, raw honey, and maple syrup

FRONTIER NATURAL PRODUCTS CO-OP
800-669-3275
frontiercoop.com
Large inventory of essential oils, base oils, organic herbs, spices, teas, dried foods and mixes, cosmetic clays, beeswax, and natural body care products

GREEN VALLEY AROMATHERAPY
877-575-7662
57aromas.com

HEAL LOCAL
heallocal.com
Medicinal herbal honey spreads, herb teas, salves, body care products, and a rose-infused honey that is divine!

HEALTHY HARVEST, LLC
healthyharvests.com
Best olive oil ever! Single estate/ varietal, organic. Exquisite facial blends and hand/foot creams.

HONEY GARDENS
800-416-2083
honeygardens.com
Raw honey, beeswax, beeswax candles, bee pollen, and delicious honey-herb blend health-promoting syrups

HYDROSOL WORLD
905-493-1572
hydrosolworld.com

JAFFE BROS.
877-975-2333
organicfruitsandnuts.com
Dried fruits, raw almond butter, seeds, beans, nuts, flours, grains, olives, spices, cereals, organic oils, prepared foods, raw honey and agave nectar, bee pollen, and organic coffee

JEAN'S GREENS HERBAL TEA WORKS & HERBAL ESSENTIALS
518-479-0471
jeansgreens.com
A wide range of wonderful herb products, teas, loose herbs and spices, essential oils, base oils, beeswax, butters, cosmetic clays, books, and more

JUST AROMATHERAPY
+44-0-782-490-5941
justaromatherapy.co.uk

KI AROMA
800-683-6739
kiaroma.ca

KING ARTHUR FLOUR COMPANY
800-827-6836
kingarthurflour.com
Fabulous flavorings, including exquisite premium vanilla and vanilla bean paste, sweet Vietnamese cinnamon, measuring tools, quality kitchen appliances and gadgets, seasonings, wheat and gluten-free flours, and more

LORANN OILS
800-862-8620
lorannoils.com
Superior-quality, concentrated, professional-strength flavorings, along with essential oils, some packaging supplies, body care crafting supplies, base oils, and candy making and baking supplies

MOUNTAIN ROSE HERBS
800-879-3337
mountainroseherbs.com
Everything you could possibly want related to herbs, plus spices, cacao powder, raw carob powder, raw cacao beans, vanilla bean powder, herb seeds, books, teas, essential and base oils, packaging supplies, herbal health aids, natural personal care products, and more

NHR ORGANIC OILS
+44-0-127-374-6505
nhrorganicoils.com

NYR ORGANIC
Stephanie Tourles, Independent Consultant/Licensed Esthetician
us.nyrorganic.com/shop/herbs
Beautiful essential oil blends and some single essential oils; exquisite organic products for skin, body, hair, and bath; herb teas; chemical-free home fragrance; heavenly organic rose and frankincense body perfumes; ultrasonic essential oil diffuser; nutritional supplements; and more

ORIGINAL SWISS AROMATICS
415-479-9120
originalswissaromatics.com
Superior-quality, therapeutic-grade essential oils derived from ethically wildcrafted or organically grown plants, along with facial, massage, and body care oils, hydrosols, and natural perfumes

PURPLE FLAME AROMATHERAPY
+44-0-167-654-2542
purpleflame.co.uk

RAW GURU
800-518-0727
rawguru.com
Raw cacao, raw foods, pure beauty-care products, and kitchen equipment for the raw foodist

SIMPLERS BOTANICALS
NutraMarks
800-229-2512
simplers.com
Superior-quality, therapeutic-grade essential oils derived from ethically wildcrafted or organically or biodynamically grown plants, along with hydrosols, perfume oils, infused herbal oils, herbal extracts, and more

SPECIALTY BOTTLE
206-382-1100
specialtybottle.com
Glass and plastic bottles, jars, and tins
of every size imaginable

STARWEST BOTANICALS
800-800-4372
starwest-botanicals.com
Essential oils, bulk herbs and spices,
teas, herbal extracts, natural body
care, packaging, and more

STILLPOINT AROMATICS
928-301-8699
stillpointaromatics.com
Exceptional-quality essential oils,
aromatherapy kits, hydrosols, flower
essences, carrier oils, infused oils,
books, and more

SUNFOOD
888-729-3663
sunfood.com
Raw foods, raw cacao, nut butters,
superfoods and supplements, books,
DVDs, pure body care products, and
kitchen appliances for the raw foodist

VOYAGEUR SOAP & CANDLE
COMPANY
800-758-7773
voyageursoapandcandle.com

Herb & Aromatherapy Education and Associations

AMERICAN COLLEGE OF HEALTHCARE
SCIENCES
800-487-8839
achs.edu
An accredited online and on-campus
college offering holistic health and
aromatherapy education

AROMAHEAD INSTITUTE
727-469-3134
aromahead.com
Online aromatherapy certification
programs, webinars on aromatherapy, body, and health care subjects,
continuing education credits, books,
and more

CANADIAN FEDERATION OF
AROMATHERAPISTS
519-746-1594
cfacanada.com

EAST-WEST SCHOOL OF PLANETARY
HERBOLOGY
800-717-5010
planetherbs.com
This school, run by Dr. Michael Tierra
and Lesley Tierra, both herbalists and
acupuncturists, offers several levels
of in-depth correspondence courses
incorporating Western, Ayurvedic, and
traditional Chinese healing systems,
plus books and Chinese herbal formulations. Highly recommended!

ESSENCE OF THYME
colleen@essenceofthyme.ca
http://essenceofthyme.ca

EVERGREEN HERB GARDEN SCHOOL
OF INTEGRATIVE HERBOLOGY
530-626-9288
evergreenherbgarden.org
An extensive herbal correspondence
course as well as local herb courses
in the High Sierra mountains of
California. These courses incorporate
Western, Ayurvedic, and Chinese
systems of herbal medicine. Highly
recommended!

HEAL LOCAL
heallocal.com
Dawn Combs teaches folkloric tradi-
tions with a contemporary knowledge
of body systems, phytochemical
compounds, and current research.
Workshops, courses, and apprentice-
ships. Highly recommended!

INTERNATIONAL FEDERATION OF
PROFESSIONAL AROMATHERAPISTS
+44-0-145-563-7987
ifparoma.org

NATIONAL ASSOCIATION FOR HOLISTIC AROMATHERAPY
919-894-0298
naha.org
An educational, nonprofit organization dedicated to enhancing public awareness, perception, and knowledge of the benefits of true aromatherapy and its safe and effective application in everyday life. NAHA maintains a listing of approved aromatherapy schools and practitioners, plus offers books, a calendar of events, and an online journal to members.

PACIFIC INSTITUTE OF AROMATHERAPY
415-479-9120
pacificinstituteofaromatherapy.com
In-depth correspondence course in French-style aromatherapy. Highly recommended!

SCHOOL OF HOLISTIC AROMATHERAPY
holisticaroma.co.uk

SCHOOL OF NATURAL HEALING
800-372-8255
snh.cc
Comprehensive herbal correspondence courses based on Western herbalism

THE SCIENCE & ART OF HERBALISM
Sage Mountain Herbal Education Center
802-479-9825
sagemountain.com
This is a lovely, in-depth, beautifully written correspondence course from herbalist Rosemary Gladstar for the beginner or intermediate-level Western herbalist. Available in either the "classic" printed version or online course. Highly recommended!

STILLPOINT STUDIES
Stillpoint Aromatics
928-301-8699
stillpointstudies.com
Excellent certification programs and workshops in aromatherapy, from beginner to advanced. Hands-on training in a classroom setting.

UNITED PLANT SAVERS
740-742-3455
unitedplantsavers.org
A nonprofit organization dedicated to conservation and cultivation of endangered native medicinal plants

WEST COAST INSTITUTE OF AROMATHERAPY
604-736-7476
westcoastaromatherapy.com

Recommended Reading

This list contains many of the resources for this book as well as selections from my personal library. If you're interested in the study of herbs, natural self-care, holistic massage therapy, essential oils and aromatherapy, and raw food nutrition, you'll find them all quite educational and enlightening.

Ackerman, Diane. *A Natural History of the Senses.* Vintage Books, 1991.

De Luca, Diana. *Botanica Erotica: Arousing Body, Mind, and Spirit.* Healing Arts Press, 1998.

Gladstar, Rosemary. *Rosemary Gladstar's Family Herbal: A Guide to Living Life with Energy, Health, and Vitality.* Storey Publishing, 2001.

———. *Rosemary Gladstar's Medicinal Herbs: A Beginner's Guide.* Storey Publishing, 2012.

Green, Mindy, and Kathi Keville. *Aromatherapy: A Complete Guide to The Healing Art.* 2nd ed. Crossing Press, 2009.

Hirsch, Alan R. *What Flavor Is Your Personality? Discover Who You Are by Looking at What You Eat.* Sourcebooks, 2001.

Inkeles, Gordon, and Murray Todris. *The Art of Sensual Massage.* Simon & Schuster, 1972.

Keville, Kathi. *Herbs: An Illustrated Encyclopedia.* Friedman/Fairfax Publishers, 1999.

Lawless, Julia. *The Encyclopedia of Essential Oils: The Complete Guide to the Use of Aromatics in Aromatherapy, Herbalism, Health & Well-Being.* Element Books, 1992.

———. *The Illustrated Encyclopedia of Essential Oils: The Complete Guide to the Use of Oil in Aromatherapy and Herbalism.* Element Books, 1995.

Maimes, Steven, and David Winston. *Adaptogens: Herbs for Strength, Stamina, and Stress Relief.* Healing Arts Press, 2007.

Miller, Bryan, and Light Miller. *Ayurveda & Aromatherapy: The Earth Essential Guide to Ancient Wisdom and Modern Healing.* Lotus Press, 1995.

Tisserand, Maggie. *Essence of Love: Fragrance, Aphrodisiacs, and Aromatherapy for Lovers.* Harper-Collins, 1993.

Tourles, Stephanie. *Hands-On Healing Remedies: 150 Recipes for Herbal Balms, Salves, Oils, Liniments & Other Topical Therapies.* Storey Publishing, 2012.

Wildwood, Chrissie. *Erotic Aromatherapy: Essential Oils for Lovers.* Sterling Publishing, 1994.

INDEX

Learn More from
BEST-SELLING HERB LOVER
Stephanie L. Tourles

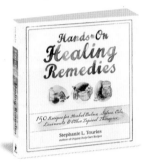

Fill your medicine cabinet with your own all-natural, topical, handmade herbal remedies. More than 100 recipes for liniments, balms, and essential oil blends will help you treat a range of ailments, from arthritis to warts.

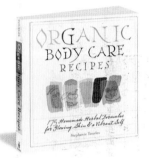

Maintain radiantly healthy and beautiful skin, hair, and body with these fun and simple recipes for creams, scrubs, toners, and much more. This wide range of beauty formulas will pamper you from head to toe with nourishing, natural ingredients.

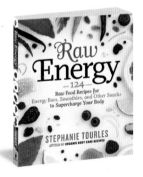

Supercharge your body with more than 100 recipes for delicious raw snacks: unprocessed, uncooked, simple, and pure. Use raw fruits, vegetables, nuts, seeds, and oils to make smoothies, trail mixes, energy bars, candies, and much more.

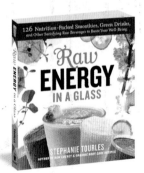

Raise a glass to longevity! Boost your health and energy using just a standard blender and these 126 super-nutritious, super-delicious recipes for smoothies, fruity frappes, vegan shakes, power shots, mocktails, and more.

These and other books from Storey Publishing are available wherever quality books are sold or by calling 800-441-5700. Visit us at storey.com or sign up for our newsletter at storey.com/signup.